BEST PRACTICES IN NURSING EDUCATION

STORIES OF EXEMPLARY TEACHERS

About the Editors

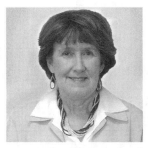

Mary Jane Smith, PhD, RN, earned her bachelor's and master's degrees from the University of Pittsburgh and her doctorate from New York University. She has been a teacher of nursing for more than a quarter of a century, at the Schools of Nursing at University of Pittsburgh, Duquesne University, Cornell University—New York Hospital, The Ohio State University, and West Virginia University. She currently holds the position of Professor and Associate Dean for Graduate Academic Affairs at West Virginia University School of Nursing.

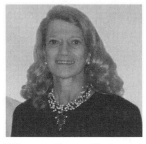

Joyce J. Fitzpatrick, PhD, RN, FAAN, earned her bachelor's degree in nursing from Georgetown University, her master's degree from The Ohio State University, and her PhD from New York University. She has also been a teacher of nursing for more than a quarter of a century, teaching at the following Schools of Nursing: Capital University, The Ohio State University, New York University, Wayne State University, Rutgers University, University of Maryland, Fairfield University, and Case Western Reserve University. She currently holds the position of Elizabeth Brooks Ford Professor of Nursing at the Frances Payne Bolton School of Nursing, Case Western Reserve University, where she was dean for 15 years.

BEST PRACTICES IN NURSING EDUCATION

STORIES OF EXEMPLARY TEACHERS

MARY JANE SMITH, PhD, RN
JOYCE J. FITZPATRICK, PhD, RN, FAAN

SP *Springer Publishing Company*

Springer Publishing Company, Inc.
11 West 42nd Street
New York, NY 10036

Acquisitions Editor: Ruth Chasek
Production Editor: Pamela Lankas
Cover design by Mimi Flow

06 07 08 09 10 / 5 4 3 2 1

Library of Congress Cataloging-in-Publication Data

Best practices in nursing education : stories of exemplary teachers / [edited by] Mary Jane Smith, Joyce J. Fitzpatrick.
    p. ; cm.
  Includes bibliographical references and index.
  ISBN 0-8261-3235-9 (soft cover)
  1. Nursing—Study and teaching. 2. Nursing schools—Faculty—Biography. 3. Nursing schools—Faculty—Vocational guidance.
    I. Smith, Mary Jane, 1938– . II. Fitzpatrick, Joyce J., 1944– .
    [DNLM: 1. Education, Nursing—Personal Narratives. 2. Faculty—Personal Narratives. WY 18 B561 2006]

RT90.B47 2006
610.73'071'1—dc22

2005012575

Printed in the United States of America by Sheridan Books Inc.

Contents

List of Tables   vii

Acknowledgments   viii

Contributors   ix

Foreword by Jeanne M. Novotny   xiv

Preface   xvii

CHAPTER   1 Introduction   1

CHAPTER   2 Diane M. Billings   3

CHAPTER   3 Rosemary Donley   9

CHAPTER   4 Florence S. Downs   20

CHAPTER   5 Vernice Ferguson   30

CHAPTER   6 M. Louise Fitzpatrick   38

CHAPTER   7 William L. Holzemer   48

CHAPTER   8 Pamela Ironside   56

CHAPTER   9 Pamela R. Jeffries   62

CHAPTER 10 Patricia R. Liehr   70

CHAPTER 11 E. Jane Martin   77

CHAPTER 12 Angela Barron McBride   87

CHAPTER 13 Diana Lynn Morris   99

CHAPTER 14 Adeline Nyamathi   107

CHAPTER 15 Marilyn Oermann   113

CHAPTER 16 Lynn Rew   118

CHAPTER 17 Grayce M. Sills   126

CHAPTER 18 Ursula Springer   134

CHAPTER 19 Christine A. Tanner   139

CHAPTER 20 Kimberly Adams Tufts   149

CHAPTER 21 Suzanne Van Ort   156

CHAPTER 22 May L. Wykle   163

CHAPTER 23 Joyce J. Fitzpatrick   171

CHAPTER 24 Mary Jane Smith   176

CHAPTER 25 Tips and Techniques for Teachers   183

Acknowledgment of Survey Participants   205

Index   207

List of Tables

TABLE 25.1 Intensive Course: Faculty Teaching Tips and Techniques   186

TABLE 25.2 Intensive Course: Students' Perspectives   187

TABLE 25.3 Clinical Course: Faculty Teaching Tips and Techniques   189

TABLE 25.4 Clinical Course: Students' Perspectives   192

TABLE 25.5 Distance Course: Faculty Teaching Tips and Techniques   195

TABLE 25.6 Distance Course: Students' Perspectives   196

TABLE 25.7 Research Course: Faculty Teaching Tips and Techniques   197

TABLE 25.8 Research Course: Students' Perspectives   199

TABLE 25.9 Meaningful Advice Given to Students by Teachers   201

Acknowledgments

We wish to acknowledge the exemplary nurse educators who so graciously participated in sharing their stories with us. We also appreciate the tips and techniques offered by faculty and students from across the United States. Names of these individuals are included in the back of the book. Special thanks to Jane Shrewsbury, for her artistic contribution with the photographs. Lastly, we wish to thank and acknowledge all of the teachers and students who the authors have had the honor to teach and learn with over the years.

MARY JANE SMITH
JOYCE J. FITZPATRICK

Contributors

Diane M. Billings, EdD, RN, FAAN, is Chancellor's Professor of Nursing and Associate Dean for Teaching, Learning, and Information Resources at Indiana University School of Nursing. She has authored nine books on nursing education, two of which received the American Journal of Nursing Book-of-the-Year Award. Dr. Billings has served as a consultant on nursing education in Jordan, Kuwait, Thailand, and the United States. She is a Fellow of the American Academy of Nursing.

Sister Rosemary Donley, PhD, RN, FAAN, is Ordinary Professor of Nursing, Director of two federally funded Community-Public Health Nursing Graduate Programs at the Catholic University of America, and First Councilor of the Sisters of Charity of Seton Hill. Sr. Rosemary is a Fellow of the American Academy of Nursing and a member of the Institute of Medicine. She was a Robert Wood Johnson Health Policy Fellow, President of the National League for Nursing, Sigma Theta Tau, and Senior Editor of *Image: The Journal of Nursing Scholarship.*

Florence S. Downs, EdD, RN, FAAN, has held significant positions in nursing, including: Professor and Director of Post-Master's Programs and Research at the Division of Nursing at New York University, Associate Dean and Professor at the University of Pennsylvania School of Nursing, and Editor of the journal *Nursing Research.* She is a Fellow of the American Academy of Nursing and was named a Living Legend of the Academy.

Vernice Ferguson, MA, RN, FAAN, was Senior Fellow in the School of Nursing at the University of Pennsylvania, holding the Fagin Family Chair in Cultural Diversity. For most of her career she has been in Federal service as the Chief Nurse at two Veterans Administration medical centers, and as Chief of the Nursing Department, Clinical Center, The National Institutes of Health. She is the recipient of eight honorary doctorates, is a Fellow in the American Academy of Nursing, and Honorary Fellow of the United Kingdom Royal College of Nursing. She was named a Living Legend of the American Academy of Nursing. Ms. Ferguson is a past president of the American Academy of Nursing, Sigma Theta Tau, and the International Society of Nurses in Cancer Care.

M. Louise Fitzpatrick, EdD, RN, FAAN, is the Connelly Endowed Dean and Professor of the College of Nursing, Villanova University. Dr. Fitzpatrick is a Fellow of the American Academy of Nursing, and has served on the Board of Governors of the National League for Nursing and American Association of Colleges of Nursing. She is past Chair of the Cabinet on Nursing Education of the American Nurses Association, and has received the National League for Nursing Award for Outstanding Leadership in Nursing Education.

William L. Holzemer, PhD, RN, FAAN, is Professor and Associate Dean for International Academic Programs in the Department of Community Health Systems, School of Nursing, University of California, San Francisco. Dr. Holzemer is a member of the Institute of Medicine, Fellow of the American Academy of Nursing, and a member of the Japan Academy of Nursing. He has edited six books and over 100 articles.

Pamela Ironside, PhD, RN, is Assistant Professor of Nursing at the University of Wisconsin-Madison. She is a member of the Board of Governors of the National League for Nursing and is a site evaluator for the Commission of Collegiate Nursing Education.

Pamela R. Jeffries, DNS, RN, is an Assistant Professor of Nursing in the Department of Adult Health at the Indiana University School of Nursing. Dr. Jeffries is Project Director of a multisite research project aimed at studying various parameters related to the use of simulation in basic nursing education programs and selected student outcomes.

Patricia R. Liehr, PhD, RN, is Professor and Associate Dean for Nursing Scholarship at Florida Atlantic University, Christine E. Lynn College of Nursing. Prior to her present role, she was Professor, Department of Theory, Research and Systems at the University of Texas Health Science Center at Houston where she was awarded the Dean's Award for Excellence in

Teaching. She is a recognized authority on middle range theory and story centered care for persons who are at risk for heart problems.

E. Jane Martin, PhD, RN, FAAN, is Professor and Dean of the School of Nursing at West Virginia University. She is a Fellow in the American Academy of Nursing and an evaluator and trainer for the Commission on Collegiate Nursing Education. She is the Dean Representative on the Accreditation Review Committee and elected Dean Representative on the CCNE Board of Commissioners. She has served as editor of the *Journal of Holistic Nursing*.

Angela Barron McBride, PhD, RN, FAAN, is a Distinguished Professor and University Dean Emerita at Indiana University School of Nursing. She is a Fellow of the American Academy of Nursing, a Distinguished Practitioner of the National Academies of Practice, and was chosen to be a National Kellogg Fellow. She has received six honorary doctorates. She is past President of Sigma Theta Tau International and the American Academy of Nursing.

Diana Lynn Morris, PhD, RN, FAAN, is an Associate Professor of Nursing and Associate Director for Programming at the University Center on Aging and Health, Case Western Reserve University. She is a Fellow in the American Academy of Nursing and is a past recipient of a National institute of Mental Health Faculty Scholar Award in Geriatric Mental Health. She has been a recipient of the National League for Nursing Lucile Petry Leone Award for Teaching Excellence, and the Elizabeth Russell Belford Founder's Award for Excellence in Education from Sigma Theta Tau.

Adeline Nyamathi, PhD, RN, FAAN, is Professor and Associate Dean for Academic Affairs at the University of California, Los Angeles School of Nursing. She is a Fellow of the American Academy of Nursing, and is responsible for organizing and implementing educational programs locally and internationally.

Marilyn Oermann, PhD, RN, FAAN, is a Professor in the College of Nursing, Wayne State University. She is the author of 10 nursing education books, some of which have received the American Journal of Nursing Book-of-the-Year Award. She is the editor of the *Annual Review of Nursing Education* and *Journal of Nursing Care Quality*. Dr. Oermann is a Fellow of the American Academy of Nursing.

Lynn Rew, EdD, RN, FAAN, is Professor, School of Nursing, University of Texas at Austin, and Director of the Southwest Partnership Center for Nursing Research on Health Disparities. She serves as the editor of the *Journal of Holistic Nursing,* and is a Fellow of the American Academy of Nursing.

Grayce M. Sills, PhD, RN, FAAN, is Professor Emeritus at the College of Nursing, The Ohio State University. She served as past president of the American Psychiatric Nurses Association and the American Nurses Foundation, and founding editor of the *Journal of the American Psychiatric Nurses Association.* She is a Fellow of the American Academy of Nursing (AAN) and has been a member of its Governing Council. She was named a Living Legend of the American Academy of Nursing.

Ursula Springer, PhD, was President of Springer Publishing Company in New York City for over 30 years. Springer specializes in publishing books for nurses, with a special focus on nursing education and research. Previously, Dr. Springer was Professor of Comparative and International Education at Brooklyn College, City University of New York. She is an honorary Fellow of the American Academy of Nursing, the Gerontological Society of America, and of Sigma Theta Tau.

Christine, A. Tanner, PhD, RN, FAAN, is the Youmann-Spaulding Distinguished Professor at the Oregon Health and Science University School of Nursing. She is a Fellow of the American Academy of Nursing. Dr. Tanner was instrumental in the founding of the Society for Research in Nursing Education. She is editor of the *Journal of Nursing Education.*

Kimberly Adams Tufts, ND, RN, FAAN, is an Associate Professor at Old Dominion University and is a Fellow of the American Academy of Nursing. She has lived and worked in Zimbabwe as a Visiting Lecturer in the Department of Nursing Science at the University of Zimbabwe.

Suzanne Van Ort, PhD, RN, FAAN, has served the College of Nursing at the University of Arizona first as a member of the faculty, then as Dean. She is a Fellow of the American Academy of Nursing, and a Fellow in the Great Britain Royal Society of Health. Dr. Van Ort has received the Sigma Theta Tau Elizabeth Russell Belford Founder's Award for Excellence in Nursing Education.

May L. Wykle, PhD, RN, FAAN, is Dean and Florence Cellar Professor of Nursing at the Frances Payne Bolton School of Nursing at Case Western Reserve University. She is a Fellow of the American Academy of Nursing and the Gerontological Society of America. She is the past President of Sigma Theta Tau International (STTI). Her awards include the STTI Elizabeth Russell Belford Founder's Award for Excellence in Nursing Education and the Lifetime Achievement Award from the National Black Nurses Association.

Foreword

I am honored to write the foreword for this book, as teaching nursing has been central to my professional life for many years. I was fascinated as I read the stories of these remarkable leaders in nursing and how they have changed the course of nursing education. The meaning of teaching and how one goes about doing it are the core subjects addressed in this book. I feel so privileged to know a number of the chapter authors, and especially to have studied with Dr. Grayce Sills during what she refers to as The Ohio State University School of Nursing's "golden era" of academic teaching.

Several themes about the nature of teaching permeate the book. Many teaching styles are described, with each having a different audience, different content, and different manner of delivery. As the contributors to the book illustrate, teaching is a personal matter, not only for the teacher, but for the learner as well. Teaching nursing is something like teaching music. You can teach someone how to play a musical instrument, but actually having that person play the instrument on their own is quite different. Successful teaching involves changing behavior in others—not an easy or always straightforward task. Moreover, many nurse educators do not view themselves first as educators, but as nurses. Nurse educators need to understand that they are part of mainstream nursing and that there is a direct correlation between what they do and how effectively the workforce is prepared. Teaching is a community activity and community property. We need to share experiences with colleagues and find time to engage in conversations with them. The contributors to this book also note that effective teaching requires ongoing feedback and evaluation systems to be in place. This is crucial to quality teaching.

Teachers should be facilitators and enablers of learning and students must be seen as partners in the learning process. Many of the personal accounts in this book discuss the nursing educators who influenced the authors' lives and made them consider a career in teaching. Often they modeled their own teaching after the good teachers in their own learning experiences.

Suggestions for enhancing comfort in a teaching role are numerous. Examples include having clear expectations and at the same time remaining flexible; remembering that comfort comes in peaks and valleys; and being passionate about one's work. In addition, content should be derived from the students' clinical experiences and the teacher should serve as a facilitator in the learning process. One should never refer to students as "my students." Instead, one should say, "They studied with me." Teaching is about presence and about who you are as a person. Teachers need to know themselves, be well grounded, have a certain confidence, and engage in reflection about their work.

In this book, the many challenges of teaching nursing are described. One common theme identified by authors is how to be a creative faculty member in a structured organization. The amount of time that faculty spend changing the curriculum is noted as taking an incredible amount of time and energy. Moreover, arguments about curriculum and what goes where can create tension among faculty.

The many rewards of teaching include the ability to influence change and to see changes in students as they develop in the nursing role. Years later, after a course is over, students often relate how much you as a teacher meant to them and what an influence you were in their lives.

I particularly like Suzanne Van Ort's description of an effective teacher, "giving the opportunity to learn, improving the ability to learn, and improving the incentive to learn. Teaching is more than covering content, teaching is opening doors, listening to students, learning with students, and being open and excited about teaching and learning." May Wykle's words of wisdom also touched me. "I have always believed that teachers ought to teach less so that students could learn more."

The teaching/learning tips and techniques offered by faculty and students will be instructive to others. The lists provided will generate dialogue among faculty colleagues and will promote the continued refinement of the process. The tips and techniques are organized within several categories, presented in the words of the faculty and students that expose the reader to the richness of the information. Students also generated a list of meaningful advice given to them by their teachers.

Best Practices in Nursing Education: Stories of Exemplary Teachers is a fascinating account of the teaching experiences of real nurse educators who have had impact on the lives of students. It is a collection of stories from the voices of 23 of the nursing profession's most experienced teachers.

This collection describes the qualities of being a nurse educator and the nature of teaching—how the act of teaching affects the lives of teachers and how it affects the lives of students. The stories serve as a source of richness and strength to both seasoned and novice teachers and will inspire nurses to select a career in which they can teach and inspire others. The cornerstones of an academic career are detailed: building collegial relationships, promoting continuous self-development, engaging in formal and informal mentoring, promoting scholarly development, and balancing professional and personal life.

This book will become a classic in the field and is a tribute to the individuals who told their stories—the stories of simple acts of everyday life, and stories of long and distinguished teaching careers. The leaders highlighted here constantly urge attention to the development of nursing education, for the purposes of transmitting knowledge to beginning and expert nurses and improving patient care.

Jeanne M. Novotny, PhD, RN, FAAN
Dean, School of Nursing
Fairfield University
Fairfield, CT

Preface

This book is written as a resource for nurse educators and as a text book for students in nursing education programs. Leading educators in graduate and undergraduate nursing programs who have demonstrated a commitment to teaching nursing tell their stories about how their teaching expertise has evolved and been sustained over time. To gather these stories we conducted personal interviews with the expert teachers, ascertaining their personal experiences as they developed their teaching expertise. Each interview and each story is unique. As authors of the book we were impressed with the stories of our colleagues and learned much from conducting the interviews. We know that you, the readers, will find the stories both instructive and entertaining, and we are indebted to our colleagues, the expert teachers, who gave generously of their time to tell us their stories. As we summarized the information obtained in the interviews we organized the stories into consistent headings for ease of use. Included in the stories are descriptions of mentoring, maintaining excellence, overcoming challenges, and advice to new teachers. These stories represent best practices in nursing education and convey an attentive concern for quality teaching, understanding of student concerns, and an energetic commitment to continuing learning for self. We believe that the reader will find these stories reassuring and enlightening. The stories illustrate that even the expert teachers among us have grown and developed through their teaching careers, often with mentoring from others, but at times, through their own initiative. Most important, the collective stories represent a perspective on nursing education that has never previously been captured for current and future nurse educators. We believe that learning from master teachers is a key strategy for preparing future generations of nurse educators.

In addition to the stories of expert teachers, lists of teaching-learning tips and techniques provided by faculty and students from across the country are included. We believe that faculty and students in nursing education programs at all levels will find the teaching tips useful in examining their own teaching. The teaching techniques that are included can be adapted for use in any nursing education setting. They will be particularly useful to new nurse educators, as they represent suggestions from both expert teachers and current students.

Collectively, the expert teachers profiled in this book have many decades of nursing education experience. We believe that future generations of nurse educators will benefit substantially from the best practices in nursing education reflected in the expert nurse educators' stories.

MARY JANE SMITH
JOYCE J. FITZPATRICK

CHAPTER 1

Introduction

Teaching is a gift that we give to each other, and learning is a gift that we give to ourselves. Teaching and learning together are as old as humankind, and the methods for explaining the process are diverse. Entire curricula in Schools of Education are devoted to the scholarship of education, and all academic disciplines engage in scholarly debates about the processes and outcomes.

This book is based on the premise that a deep storehouse of knowledge resides in the stories of experienced teachers. This knowledge is often transmitted on a one-to-one basis, from mentor to mentee, but otherwise lies hidden until accessed through gathering the stories of experiences, ideas, and actions of teachers. The stories that follow flowed from interviews conducted with 21 teachers at various levels in their career. The participants were engaged in a conversation with us and asked to talk about the following: how their teaching expertise had evolved and been sustained over time, how they decided on a career in teaching nursing, how they were prepared and mentored in teaching, how they maintained excellence, when they felt comfortable as a teacher, the most and least rewarding times in teaching, embarrassing teaching moments, significant challenges, and lastly, advice for new teachers. We found the teachers we interviewed to be quite engaged in telling their stories. They were enlivened as they moved in and through the recollections of their story of teaching. At the end of the conversation they expressed that participation was enjoyable and valuable. These stories are testimonies to the power of story to create meaning.

We selected individuals for interviews based on our personal experiences with them as teachers and mentors, because we were aware of their current stature in the nursing education community of scholars, or because they had been recipients of national teaching awards. Everyone invited was eager to participate in the interview and to tell their story.

Hearing the voice of these experienced teachers can help other faculty as they take on the role of teacher in an academic setting. Stories lead us into the lives of those who have been there, by offering connections with the issues, expectations, fears, and joys that come with living the life of teacher. In making the connections, insights are gleaned and steps along the way are made concrete. Considering how others have integrated the role of teacher into their lives may offer support that goes beyond the usual activities of faculty development.

Embedded in the stories are tried and tested practices of teaching, including building collegial relationships, continuous self-development, formal and informal mentoring, scholarly development, and balancing professional and personal life. Each story is unique, demonstrating both the patterns in leadership development and the individual manner in which experts make their way in the professional world of leaders. Some of the experiences no doubt reflect the times; for example, becoming a leader in nursing education in the 1960s is a bit different than leadership development in 2005. Yet, the similarities also are remarkable, as nursing continues to evolve as an academic discipline.

The final two stories were written by the editors of the book. Based on our commitment to excellence in nursing education, the raison d'etre for this book, we thought it was important to share our own development and evolution as nurse educators. We stand among giants, though, the 21 others' profiles preceding our own.

Chapter 25 includes the results of a survey that was conducted among contemporary teachers and students in nursing at several schools within the editors' range of contact. Participation was completely voluntary and conducted by colleagues through distribution of questionnaires. We aimed for representation in a number of different teaching formats, such as distance education courses, and courses that were either primarily didactic or clinical in focus. Teachers and students shared their comments openly. We are indebted to all of these participants and have acknowledged them at the end of the book.

Finally, this book will serve as an historical document, charting the contributions of these expert teachers in nursing education in the last half century in the United States. We believe that the best practices in teaching/learning are grounded in the stories of these dedicated teachers and students living the experience. It is expected that these stories will generate enthusiasm and spark a deepened commitment to the life project of teaching and learning.

CHAPTER 2

Diane M. Billings

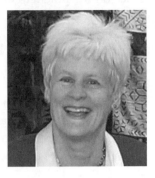

BACKGROUND

Diane M. Billings is Chancellor's Professor of Nursing and Associate Dean for Teaching, Learning and Information Resources at Indiana University School of Nursing. In this role she is responsible for the Center for Teaching and Lifelong Learning, Continuing Nursing Education, Learning Resource Center, Distance Learning Programs and Faculty and Staff Information Resources. She earned a BSN from Duke University, MSEd from Butler University, and EdD from Indiana University.

Dr. Billings is a Fellow in the American Academy of Nursing and was awarded the Elizabeth Russell Belford Founder's Award for Excellence in Education, Sigma Theta Tau International. She received the Excellence in Educational Technology Award from the National Nursing Staff Development Organization, and was a Mira Award Finalist for the innovative use of information technology to improve public health.

Dr. Billings has authored nine books on nursing education; two of these received the American Journal of Nursing Book of the Year Award. In addition she has written numerous book chapters and published over 50 articles on education. She has served as a consultant on nursing education in Jordan, Kuwait, Thailand, and the United States.

STORY INTRODUCTION

Dr. Billings believes that a teacher should not have a goal of being in charge of the classroom, rather she or he should aim to be a facilitator and enabler of student learning. She guides faculty to embrace the full faculty role in the academic setting by developing new knowledge and disseminating evidence on the practices of teaching and learning.

EARLY INTEREST IN TEACHING

I do not know that I ever set out precisely to be a teacher. I was about a year into a staff nurse position in a public health department, and one of the faculty from Indiana University School of Nursing asked me to teach a postconference to her students. I absolutely loved it. I loved preparing and working with the students. It opened a whole new avenue to me. Then, that faculty member recommended me for a teaching position at a diploma school in Indianapolis. I pursued it, and that is how I got started as a teacher.

Back then, a diploma school was a good environment to start a teaching career because it was a small program, there were a lot of experienced teachers, and the focus was on the student. Faculty were an integral part of the student's life. Furthermore, the program was really connected to clinical practice. What we were teaching in the classroom was immediately applied to practice in the hospital. All students were at the same hospital and we knew what was going on there. It was a nice, easy way to start teaching, and ever since I have loved it. This was in 1966. I started out my teaching very early, with 2 years of staff nurse experience. Shortly thereafter, the diploma program closed and became connected with the Purdue Associate Degree program, which, at that time, was an extension in Indianapolis. I taught at the Purdue program for about 3 months when there was a merger between Indiana University and Purdue University in Indianapolis. The question at that historical moment was, what to do with nursing in the Indiana system? Should we have a separate associate degree program located in the school of liberal arts or should the associate degree program be in the School of Nursing, where the baccalaureate, master's, and doctoral programs resided? Dean Emily Holmquist was able to unite all the programs back into one school, and this is how I became a faculty member at Indiana University School of Nursing.

PREPARATION FOR TEACHING

My early teaching probably involved repeating some of the things I saw my own teachers do. However, I could see immediately that I did not have enough background or preparation for teaching. So, I earned a master's degree in education from Butler University, because at the time, I was not aware of any nursing schools who were really preparing faculty, and the program at Butler prepared professionals for the teaching role. I loved all of the courses and it all seemed so natural. I was able to apply the content of the courses that I was taking to the teaching that I was doing. Other preparation came from attending workshops, watching other faculty, and trying things out in a kind of trial and error way. In my doctoral program, I focused on education with a degree in instructional technology, which I earned in 1986. That educational preparation helped me form my current position as Associate Dean of Teaching, Learning and Information Resources.

Soon after I went to Purdue, we were teaching an integrated curriculum, but all of the textbooks were written for the segregated curriculum. Lillian Stokes, Janet Barber, and I had the idea that we needed a better textbook for the integrated associated degree programs. A major publisher quickly signed the three young faculty and that book lasted for four editions. From this experience, I learned that writing textbooks really is another way of teaching, probably at a more global level than classroom teaching.

MENTORING FOR TEACHING

When I first started teaching I was mentored by some experienced teachers and the Director of the Diploma Program. I think that she could see that I had potential and she went out of her way to keep tabs on what I was doing. I could go in and talk to her and she would give me advice. Back then the mentor role was probably never identified as it is today. People did not even take it upon themselves to recognize that someone needed a mentor and then offered to do it. Later on in my career, Angela McBride and Rebecca Markle were mentors. What I think was happening then, and I see it now because I am a mentor, is that a lot of mentoring happens behind the scenes. I can now reflect back and see that somebody said, "Let's ask Diane to do it." or, "Let's give her a chance to work on this project in this area." Mentoring is making opportunities available, or making them happen. I think probably more of that went on than I am aware of; where a teacher's life is touched by somebody who is in the background as mentor.

EVOLUTION AS A TEACHER

I am always evolving as a teacher because the students have changed, and we are always trying to be responsive to their needs. My teaching has also changed and evolved because of the learning resources that are available. The best example here is the computer technology course that I have taught for 12 years. This one course has had major revisions each year because the technology that is discussed in the course has changed so much. My teaching has evolved because of my response to curricular changes over the years and because of things that I learned as I integrate new ways of being and doing into my teaching practices.

FEELING COMFORTABLE AS A TEACHER

I don't know that I am ever totally comfortable as a teacher. Comfortableness comes in peaks and in valleys. For example, when I moved from the associate degree program to the baccalaureate program, I was a novice teacher again. You start all over and have to rethink the curriculum and the level of students. Each time you make a major change to another level, it takes a little while to get comfortable. One change that is happening to most educators now, is moving from the traditional classroom to the on-line environment. I believe this change makes faculty uncomfortable because as experienced teachers they end up being novices again. There are always changes. I think it is this part that makes it fun, you do not get stagnant.

CHALLENGES AS A TEACHER

I think the biggest challenge comes with being a creative faculty member within a structured organization. When the structure is rigid and when colleagues do not understand what you are doing, it is a challenge to maintain creativity. I give credit to Dean Angela McBride for understanding creativity and not restricting my creativity or that of anyone else. Thus, challenge came in trying to figure out how the organizational structure fit with my skills and interests.

Introducing technology into the curriculum also created some challenges. Bringing people along was a challenge. My role at that time was not just to integrate technology into my own teaching, but to try to help educators at my own school and anyone else who was interested and wanted to come along.

EMBARRASSING TEACHING MOMENTS

I cannot pull anything funny or embarrassing out of my memory that sticks with me. I am sure there were many, but nothing comes to mind.

REWARDING ASPECTS OF TEACHING

Teaching in an environment where the opportunity to move, influence change, and push the envelope is rewarding. The most rewarding period of my career has been the last 10 years because things have come together. The evolution of a teacher takes time because there are many things that need to be developed and unfold over a period of time. Earning advanced degrees to support what you are doing kind of diverts some energy away from what you can do because you have to be focused on learning how to do it. It all came together after I earned my doctoral degree and had the opportunity to work in broader environments than in the classroom. However, seeing people learn or do something that was believed to be impossible is the most rewarding of all, and that aspect of teaching transcends all changes in curriculum or technology.

LEAST REWARDING ASPECTS OF TEACHING

The least rewarding time in my career was when I was working in an environment where the organizational structure, the political structure, and the administrative structure was very rigid. During some of these times, we were coming out of that diploma school-teaching model, and not everyone understood the faculty role in a university setting that was more than just the teaching. The role included scholarship, service, and research. When the environment did not support the full faculty role, that for me was extremely frustrating.

MAINTAINING EXCELLENCE AS A TEACHER

I go to conferences. I work with other people and see how they are doing things. I read a lot. I keep trying to test new ideas. If something is coming along, I will see what it takes to do it, and try it. My courses are always being revised. I like to see how they work for the students and then revise accordingly. Feedback from students is key to identifying what is working and what is not. I go out and talk to people and get new ideas that I bring to my teaching.

ADVICE FOR NEW TEACHERS

I think new teachers should be prepared for the role, listen to the students, and be student centered. New teachers should see their role as a facilitator of student learning. I think a lot of faculty, old and new, still see themselves as being the one who is in charge and in control. As we move into the future, this is not going to be the faculty role. I would tell new teachers that they should not go down that path of trying to be in charge of a classroom. Rather, they should be a facilitator and enabler of student learning. They should try to understand that their role is broader than just teaching. Their role in the academic institution is the development of new knowledge and the dissemination of best practices about teaching and learning. New teachers should get involved and get focused in their teaching/learning practices, find what they like to do, and then do it well. Above all, be themselves, be true to their own values, and be real with students.

CHAPTER 3

Rosemary Donley

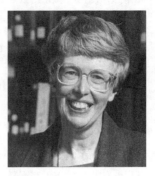

BACKGROUND

Sister Rosemary Donley is an Ordinary Professor of Nursing, Director of two federally funded Community/Public Health Nursing Graduate Programs at The Catholic University of America, Washington, D.C., and First Councilor of the Sisters of Charity of Seton Hill. Sr. Rosemary received a diploma from the Pittsburgh Hospital School of Nursing and holds a BSN summa cum laude from St. Louis University and a MNEd and PhD from the University of Pittsburgh. She is a certified adult nurse practitioner. Her clinical and research interests are health policy, clinical decision making, and health care literacy.

Sr. Rosemary is a Fellow in the American Academy of Nursing and a member of the Institute of Medicine. She was a Robert Wood Johnson Health Policy Fellow, past President of the National League for Nursing, Sigma Theta Tau International Honor Society of Nursing, and Senior Editor of *Image: The Journal of Nursing Scholarship*. She has over 90 publications and has presented papers throughout the United States and abroad.

STORY INTRODUCTION

Sr. Rosemary Donley has dedicated her life to improving the quality of health care. Her early entry into teaching was motivated by the belief that she could do more to raise the quality of care through educating students. Her life as a teacher has been shaped by her religious community

9

and educational preparation in higher education, administration, psychiatric mental health nursing, health policy analysis, and most recently in advanced nursing practice as a family nurse practitioner.

EARLY INTEREST IN TEACHING

I had just begun nursing in a diploma school in the early 1960s and another nun and I met with our superior. I do not remember exactly what she said; it was something about how it takes 5 or 6 years of education to produce a teacher or supervisor. The next time I thought about teaching was when I was finishing the diploma program. In my senior year I had another conversation with the superior and she asked me about teaching. She told me that in a religious community, you were a nurse, a teacher, or perhaps an administrator. I thought what she was saying to me was that the community was going to take me from nursing and place me in a teaching position in elementary school. I told her that I loved nursing, and did not want to be a teacher. "Oh, no, no, no," she said. "We are talking about teaching nursing—do you think you would like that?" So very quickly that afternoon, I told her I had never thought of it, but perhaps I would like to be a teacher of nursing. She indicated that they were talking about where they were going to send me to school to get my baccalaureate degree. It dawned on me that I was being told I was going to be prepared to be a teacher. I thought if I were a teacher, I could raise the standards, raise the bar, and improve the quality of care for others much better than if I were a staff nurse. I knew I wanted to be a teacher when I realized I could improve the quality of care as a teacher beyond what I could do myself.

PREPARATION FOR TEACHING

I went to St. Louis University knowing that I was being prepared to be a nurse educator. After graduation I was assigned to be an assistant teacher in fundamentals of nursing in the diploma program from which I graduated. At the same time I began the master's degree program in medical nursing at the University of Pittsburgh. One of the faculty, Dr. Lois Austin, knew a lot about education and taught a number of courses on curriculum and evaluation. Plus there were clinical courses and practice teaching courses. While in the master's program I was teaching in a diploma school. I was now teaching some of the things I was learning. I completed the master's program in December 1965, right after Medicare was enacted. I remember thinking that the students had no understanding of Medicare. So I found someone in the business office to teach Medicare even though he could not understand why nurses needed to know about Medicare. I thought they did and I still think so.

Shortly after this, the psychiatric hospital where students affiliated was undergoing some changes and they needed teachers. I was asked if I would like to teach psychiatric nursing. I had just finished my master's degree in medical nursing, and could see how an understanding of medical nursing and chronic illness was related to emotional and mental health. So I went back to the University of Pittsburgh to study again. It turned out that there was a joint program with the psychiatric hospital to prepare people in education and service in acute care hospitals to learn about adjustment and psychiatric disorders, disguised or presented as medical or surgical. I was told that if I could find someone from my institution in nursing service willing to attend we could begin this wonderful program. I went to my community, found a partner in administration and attended the 9-month program. Anthropologists, nurses, psychiatrists, and persons with public/health/social science backgrounds taught the courses. It was a wonderful learning experience but I thought I needed clinical experience. A special program was worked out for me on a private floor at Western Psychiatric Institute, because the patients there stayed a little longer and I was interested in psychotic disorders. One day I got a message that one of the psychiatrists wanted to see me; he talked to me for a while and said that he wanted to make a deal with me. He would supervise me if I would be the primary therapist with one of his in-patients. I told him that I did not know enough to do that. He indicated the man was quite ill, and that I was the only one to whom he was talking. I asked how he knew he was talking to me. He responded that the nurses said that I had come out of his room and told them he had terrible laryngitis, a fever, and needed some treatment. Because of how he was acting, they just did not go near him. So, I worked in this capacity for about 3 years. Then, I went to Columbia University in the summers and took courses in psychiatric nursing. I then began to teach psychiatric nursing and work with students in a community mental health unit at St. Frances Hospital. It was a good place for students as they saw good models of nursing and team practice.

One of the faculty at the University of Pittsburgh's School of Public Health, Dr. Ahlon Shiloh, told me I should go on and get a doctorate. He said I was bright and needed credentials. At that point, the University of Pittsburgh was only offering doctorates in maternal child health nursing.

Dr. George Fahey (Professor of Educational Psychology) and Dr. Shiloh worked out a program where I would do part of my work in the Graduate School of Public Health, and part of my work in higher education, all at the University of Pittsburgh. Because I taught psychiatric nursing in a 9-week term I could schedule classes full time in the doctoral program. I finished the class work in 1969, and wrote my dissertation in 1971.

EVOLUTION AS A TEACHER

I then received a call from the University of Pittsburgh telling me that Dr. Lois Austin was retiring and that she recommended that I take over her courses. I told them that I was her student and was not sure that I was good enough to teach her courses. Yet I assumed the position and ended up teaching the education courses the next year. At the end of the year, I was offered two full-time positions at Pitt. One was as chair of medical surgical nursing and the other was a faculty appointment in general nursing, which would include teaching education courses. The person in charge, Alice Malone, had been given authority to hire faculty to do nothing but plan a graduate program to prepare educators and administrators. I went back and forth and thought I was not ready to be in charge of the medical surgical nursing. It was not teaching. I could teach medical surgical nursing but was not prepared to be responsible for a department. So, I took the position in general nursing.

I was happy at Pitt teaching graduate students. We built the program. The program was very popular because we taught in the late afternoon. Alice Malone, who was in charge of the program, was one smart lady. She protected the faculty. She made sure we had what we needed, and this was probably the best first teaching position one could have in a university. She mentored me in that she showed me the right way to do things. She brought in consultants to help us and treated us with great respect. I was young, just 23 or 24 years old. She was very proud of our work. She recognized that junior faculty in an academic hierarchy are at the bottom and somebody needs to be for them and so she was incredibly supportive of us. We could always go and talk to her about a problem student or a problem situation and she would give good advice. She could also intervene. There were a lot of kingdoms, and she was able to work through the kingdoms to get a program approved. She provided me with an experience of what the faculty role should be in a nursing school. I was there 8 years. I was too young to realize this was not the universal faculty experience. It is only later that I have seen that. Alice Malone encouraged me and helped me apply for tenure. I was tenured early at the University of Pittsburgh. When we were doing things that were not appropriate, she would tell us. She would say the timing is not right with this. She would call us "kids"; and, one of the "kids" was in her sixties. She formed a group and we met at least every week. We really knew what was going on in the University and in the School. She was a wonderful mentor, is still alive, and I keep in touch with her.

During this time, I was preparing teachers and taught courses in role development, trends and issues, along with clinical teaching. Teaching the trends and issues was how I got into policy. I began to see that it did not matter what text or frame of reference you used, nursing always had the same problems.

One day, Dr. Robert Hickey, an assistant to the Vice Chancellor for Health, asked me if I knew about the Robert Wood Johnson Health Policy Fellowship. I picked up an application and was told that the university was going to nominate a faculty member and that they would provide help completing the application. It was due in 5 days. With help, the application was put together and I was invited to be interviewed and was later selected as a 1977–1978 Fellow, the second nurse fellow.

After a year on the hill, my teaching changed again because I could really see the role of policy and its influence on quality of care and nursing practice. I have taught health policy ever since; it is particularly critical with chronic illness, and for people with physical and mental disabilities. Dr. Hickey and Nathan Stark, the Vice Chancellor, are deceased. I credit them for my opportunity to learn policy. While I was in Washington, D.C., with the Fellowship, the President, Dr. Clarence Walton, opened the search for Dean at The Catholic University of America and they asked me to be a consultant for the search process. I was not interested in being a dean. I was very happy with what I was doing in Pittsburgh. However, they kept persuading and persuading me until everybody was annoyed with me for not making the decision. I finally ended up saying that I would assume the dean role, and that is how I got to The Catholic University of America (CUA) in 1979. As Dean, I continued to teach every semester. Along with my teaching responsibilities, I had other responsibilities to the students and faculty. I tried to figure out ways around the University system so that faculty without doctorates could earn doctoral degrees and worked to develop an environment where scholarship flourished. Dr. Edmund Pellegrino, a physician, succeeded Clarence Walton as President of CUA and was instrumental in my assuming the dean role. However he left the University at the end of my second year as Dean. We had a very good working relationship and I was disappointed that he was leaving. A nurse colleague said to me, "What makes you think the new president won't be better?" I never thought of it that way. So, through a democratic process, I was elected to serve on the Presidential search committee. I met the candidates and participated in the selection of the new president. I was happy being Dean and liked it. It was one of the nicest positions I have ever had.

In 1984 President William J. Byron, S. J., asked me to take the role of Executive Vice President. This was very difficult because I was a woman and this was a university run by men. So I was mentored by the then Executive Vice President, Dr. John Murphy, and later went to Harvard's executive training program. In the fall of 1986, I took on the responsibility. During this time I continued to teach one course a year. As Executive Vice President, or Chief Operating Officer, my time was not my own. Five vice presidents and several departments reported to me. I had budgetary responsibility, and could always be sure that the academic environment got its fair share. Even though I did not totally understand informational technology, I made the decision to wire the entire campus. I had no scientific insights into the information age, but it felt right. CUA was one of the first campuses that was completely wired. We worked to get all the faculty and students access to computers and to learn or sharpen their computer skills. During the Byron years, CUA was engaged in a $100 million capital campaign. I learned something about fund-raising. I had a very good working relationship with the President. We never played power games with each other and he never disagreed with any decision I made.

During the presidency of Brother Patrick Ellis, FSC, I was elected to be one of my religious community's general superiors. The election was a surprise. I knew one day that I was going to be asked to help the Sisters of Charity of Seton Hill. However, I also knew that holding two positions was problematic. The major superior, Sr. Gertrude Foley, wanted me to be in Greensburg, PA full time. Under these circumstances, I knew that I could not be Executive Vice President. You had to be available; you could not be away. Sr. Gertrude understood my love for nursing. She told me that I could teach nursing if I agreed to return to Greensburg each week for several days. So I began the 10-hour round-trip commute each week. I would leave the University Thursday afternoon and be back on campus Tuesday. So, I resigned my administrative position, finished out the year, and began my term as general councilor in June 1997.

After finishing my university administrative tour, I had a sabbatical, which was wonderful. I decided that if I were going to get back into nursing as a teacher, I better get caught up. I had not practiced for some time and so I did what I always do when I need to learn something. I went back to school and became an Adult Nurse Practitioner. Everybody thought I was crazy. I really was interested in learning how managed care affects nursing practice and health care delivery. That was why I became a nurse practitioner. I wanted to see how health care delivery was changed by managed care. I would use the practitioner education as a way of looking at the care. I finished the program, and came back to teach full time. Currently, I also teach policy to doctoral and master's students, courses in population health, and a course in health promotion, which I love. I direct three federally funded master's level programs in care of vulnerable people. One program prepares clinical specialists in community/public health nursing; another, family nurse practitioners and community/public health specialists for a blended role; and a third prepares teachers of community/public health nursing. Here in Washington, people are now interested in the public health infrastructure. The District provides many examples of failures in the health infrastructure such as lead in the water.

FEELING COMFORTABLE AS A TEACHER

I felt comfortable in the role of teacher when I completed the Fellowship and had a good understanding of health policy. Nineteen seventy-seven to seventy-eight was a wonderful year to learn policy. I still reach back to that. I think because it was so focused, it helped me shape what I was doing, and was going to do. So the Fellowship that helped me as a teacher changed my professional life. It gave me some direction. It probably took me away from some other things, because that is what a focus does.

CHALLENGES AS A TEACHER

I never planned to be an administrator, and I told myself that what I was trying to do as Dean of Nursing at The Catholic University of America, was not real administration; but when I became Executive Vice President, I could not say that. On leaving administration, I questioned whether I could come back and teach again. Could I teach the advanced practice of nursing? Could I get myself up to speed again? The answer is yes and no. Six years later . . . I am aware that I will never be the clinician I was in 1979. The skills came back, but the clinical judgment required of a nurse practitioner in primary care is different. I found out that I did not know enough and that if I were actually going to be a good nurse practitioner, I would be reading and taking continuing education workshops every weekend; I also have limited my practice to something in which I have an interest, chronically ill people.

REWARDING ASPECTS OF TEACHING

When I first came back to teach, I asked if I could teach foundations of nursing, which is where I started many years ago. To watch students learn assessment skills at the beginning of the semester and see them develop so that they are organized and have some sense of professional behavior is rewarding. I think rewards come when a student actually changes and you can see change. I do not mean changes on test scores. You can actually see real change, when you talk to students or read their logs and papers. You can see critical analysis, better use of the literature, better ideas, and sometimes creative ideas. I enjoy seeing students putting it together. I keep in touch with students, which takes time and energy, but it is nice to see what they are doing and how they have developed their lives.

LEAST REWARDING ASPECTS OF TEACHING

It is not rewarding when there are barriers in the system, particularly when these barriers create problems for students. For example, we are registering students right now. There was a lack of care in developing course scheduling, which is a central administrative function. Incompetence drives me crazy.

I find the lack of appreciation of diversity difficult to accept. Some faculty want the students to be all the same. In our community/public health programs, 70% of our students are from diverse backgrounds. We have intentionally recruited culturally diverse and minority nurses. When they come back to school, some of them do not know how to use computers for anything but fill in blanks. So, there is a lot of work to help them learn skills that graduate students need. I find this very exciting. They are a wonderful group to work with and they have a broad base of experience. The dialogue and discussion is just amazing. I find that very exciting. I do not like homogenization. I guess to synthesize what is least rewarding for me, it is a lack of appreciation that the workforce of the future is not going to be like the workforce of the past. Each teacher has to reinvent herself or himself. You have to figure out how to teach today's students.

EMBARRASSING TEACHING MOMENTS

I have a sense of humor, so there probably are a lot of funny ones. I do not get embarrassed, at all, if the Power Points do not work. I turn them off and write on the board. I once had an experience where I brought the wrong paper to a lecture in another city. This was very interesting because I had to reconstruct a paper from my head. I don't know whether that was embarrassing or funny, but I told the people what happened and asked for their patience.

I have two nightmares. In the first nightmare, I go to the wrong city to give a paper, or I go the wrong day, so I have place/time confusion. The other nightmare is, I get to the right place but I do not have the right paper or the latest version of the paper. I have often wondered what I would do when that happened. It did. I made a little outline and told the audience that I was worried about keeping to the time. I usually know what I am talking about. However, my sentence structure was rambling at times and I was worried about the time. This experience was not funny and it was not embarrassing. It called me to reexamine my lifestyle. I asked myself, are you too busy, what are you doing? I tend to be introspective. So, it was a clue to me that maybe things were going too fast.

MAINTAINING EXCELLENCE AS A TEACHER

You have to reinvent yourself. I do not know how many times you have to do it, but you have to keep reinventing yourself. If you're teaching in a clinical world or policy world, you have to keep up with it. Keeping up is reading, and writing, because you learn when you write. It is doing research. It is periodically stopping and actually going back to school formally. I have always been able to go back to school. I also learn from students. I learn from the preceptors. I learn from patients. I learn from my colleagues on the faculty; but I think if you want to be a teacher, you have to be 5 or 10 years ahead of where the field is. I probably take teaching for the future too seriously. Reinventing yourself means you volunteer to teach something that you have not taught before. I keep struggling for a better way to present a course to the students, so that it makes sense. I am not the teacher who goes into the computer and pulls up and then modifies material. I am always changing the class content. Maybe I change it too much. I think the commitment to excellence, and the commitment to scholarship, is a commitment to keep learning. At CUA, we say the faculty and students are a community of scholars, and I take that seriously.

It is a community of scholars so you are not out there by yourself. What you're doing is working toward some kind of common good. At least this is my interpretation of a community of scholars. Teaching is about scholarship. It is not about one-up-man-ship. It is about interpreting a body of knowledge or contributing to it. It is about knowledge development and knowledge expansion. You are a member of the community because you are a teacher of people who are going to come after you, that's another communal dimension. The students are part of the community, so you are to be a learner with the students, not lording it over them. Teachers are supposed to learn with students and from them. You appreciate and respect the students and your colleagues in this endeavor.

ADVICE FOR NEW TEACHERS

New teachers should select a good school for their first position. Pick a school where somebody has time for you—it may not be the Dean, but, maybe somewhere in the environment, there is an Alice Malone. Work on what you are doing. There are some people who do not like teaching, and if that is so, do not try to do something you do not like. Find a university or college where the environment fits you. You may not have to know the people there, but you have to believe in what they are doing, and how they see their work. In the beginning, new teachers need help with clinical evaluations, paper evaluations, and writing tests. New teachers have to do a lot of learning on their own. So, it is important to find a good school that values teaching for your first job. New teachers with a PhD have so many things to do, because they are under the tenure constraint. They have to start to pursue a research agenda, publish, and also learn to teach. Most master's prepared nurses are coming out of practitioner programs. They teach undergraduate students with very different domains of knowledge. That is an adjustment.

I look at teaching as changing behavior. If I were to pick a book to recommend it would be something about change theory. It might be some of the work by deClememte, who talks about changing behavior. I do not know if I necessarily read books on teaching. I probably did at one point, when I was in my master's program, but I have not read many since. I would say if you are going to teach something, know your subject, because the method flows from the subject.

For example, when I began to teach population-based health care, I had to study what it was about and how to assess communities. I had to look at all the models on population assessment. I had to decide which ones made most sense to me. I began to talk about vulnerability. I did a lot of reading on vulnerability, and how to assess a population or a person for vulnerability. That is how I prepare to teach. I immerse myself into content, from a wide range of sources. I also read the nursing authors, but I read a very, very wide range of authors. I spent half my life studying to teach. I literally prepare for every class.

CHAPTER 4

Florence S. Downs

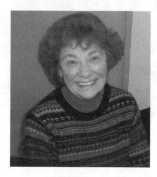

BACKGROUND

Dr. Florence S. Downs holds a diploma in nursing from St. Luke's Hospital School of Nursing, a BS from St. Johns University, and an MA and EdD from New York University. She has held significant positions in nursing including: Professor and Director of Post-Master's Programs and Research at the Division of Nursing at New York University, Professor and Associate Dean and Director of Graduate Studies at the University of Pennsylvania School of Nursing, and Editor of *Nursing Research*. Most recently, she was a Visiting Scholar at University of Pennsylvania School of Nursing; Division of Nursing, New York University; and University of Maryland School of Nursing.

Dr. Downs was a member of the groups that initiated the Council of Nurse Researchers and the Eastern Nursing Research Society. Throughout her academic career she has taught research design and dissertation seminars. She chaired the committees of 102 doctoral students and served as a member of innumerable others. She is widely published including works in research journals, books, and editorials.

STORY INTRODUCTION

A significant part of Dr. Downs's career as an educator has been as a teacher of research and mentor to doctoral students in nursing. She believes that teaching is more of an art than a science and that students learn when the teacher touches their experience in a meaningful way. She views herself as having had a long and happy life as an educator.

EARLY INTEREST IN TEACHING

I knew the exact moment when it first occurred to me that I wanted to be a teacher. I had joined the New York City public health department to be a public health nurse. At a training program there was a nutritionist providing a class on the topic of what a person should eat. I recall thinking, "Oh no, nutrition again"; since of course, I already knew a lot about nutrition. However, this teacher was great as she lectured and cooked many different dishes. I tasted some of these foods for the first time and thought they were really great. At this time I said to myself: "Wouldn't it be wonderful if I could be a teacher and help change people's minds." I remember this just like it was yesterday.

PREPARATION FOR TEACHING

When I was at NYU, there was an argument about whether I should take the EdD or the PhD. I went back and forth and re-matriculated three times. In the course of re-matriculating, I took all the courses for both degrees and wound up with 105 credits above the baccalaureate. The maximum needed was 96. I took courses in curriculum instruction, apprentice college teaching, and other how-to-teach courses. I do not think these courses helped me very much. I did learn how to organize the subject matter in a course and how to divide it up in sections; but to teach is more art than science. A person can be taught to use Power Point slides but that is not really teaching. Teaching is getting to the students and digging out from them what they need to absorb in order for them to get what it is you want them to learn, and most importantly, for the students to learn the content in a way that they can use. I think some of how teachers teach is a matter of personality. An approach could be suggested to you and you would say, "Oh, Florence! I couldn't do that." If it does not fit the teacher's way of doing things then it will not work. Teaching is a Sarah Bernhardt thing and that is the hardest part. Teachers can be taught to organize, set up objectives, and all of the other kinds of structured teaching techniques; but to get the material across to students is another story entirely. For me, it was trial and error. Had I really learned how to teach would I have had stage fright? Probably not.

Now in many doctoral programs they say, "Well, nobody teaches you how to teach." So, they have these various teaching courses including apprentice teaching, and one of the points that always comes up is that some of the doctoral students have been teaching students for years and know how to teach. I believe there are many kinds of teaching. Each kind of teaching has a different audience, different content, and different ways that are probably the best way to deliver content. For a long time, for instance, in the clinical situations, nurses used audio or videos to teach patients. They would say, "We don't have to waste our time teaching, show patients a video and they can learn from it." I question if this approach is as good as having somebody with you, talking about it, and pacing learning to what can be absorbed at the time. I think teaching is such a personal matter, not only for the teacher, but also for the learner and the content. There are lectures, small groups, and one-on-one modes. Each requires a very different approach. I believe a person cannot know what it is like until they do it. It is something like teaching poker. You can teach somebody how to play poker, but actually playing poker is very different.

MENTORING FOR TEACHING ROLE

I cannot recall any mentor who helped me with teaching.

EVOLUTION AS A TEACHER

I was in the psychiatric nursing program at New York University, had completed the master's work, and was working on my doctorate, in a program that went from bachelor's to doctorate. After I had completed all the psychiatric nursing work, they wanted me to teach in the program, that is how I began my teaching career. The course consisted entirely of seminars and one-on-one meetings with the students. Martha Rogers was anxious for me to finish the doctoral program because I was not supposed to be teaching graduate students with just a baccalaureate degree. Therefore, I had to be kept undercover at all times.

Teaching a Lecture Course

Once I earned my doctorate, I continued to teach in the psychiatric nursing program until Martha Rogers decided that I should be teaching research. I was delighted to teach research because I thought I really knew all about research since, after all, I did have a doctorate. In the psychiatric nursing program, the teaching modalities that I had used were small group seminars and the one-on-one interactions. However, in the research class there were about 75 students. In those days we did not have teaching assistants. It was a big deal to have 75 students in a class. I prepared all of the lessons, walked into the classroom, stepped up on the platform, and got the worse case of the shakes that I have ever had. I was scared witless, proceeded to talk, and then covered the whole course in one night. I went back to the office, sat in the chair, and thought, "What am I going to do? I taught it all!" After calming down, I decided to tell the students that the first class was an overview of the course and that I would proceed with more precision thereafter. After a while I did get used to teaching large groups of students and became a Sarah Bernhardt. This is what one really needs to do, in order to teach a lecture course well. I believe you have to be able to get something back from the student; it is just like being an actress. As a teacher, you get vibes from the students in the audience and you know when they are with you, and when they are not with you. When they are not with you, you feel sort of defeated. This staying with the students takes really hard work. The teacher has to understand what kinds of things will hold the students' attention, and doing this is not something that can be taught. It is something teachers have to learn by experience. Having a good sense of humor helps a lot. I learned to do all kinds of things that were related to the students' experiences. One of the things I used to do was to use two sets of dice. One set was loaded. I would have the students shoot the dice to make sample selections in order to teach them the nature of bias and what could happen to the sample if biased subjects were chosen. I always tried to keep the students with me. I gave them a semantic differential about research at the beginning of the course and another at the end of the course to help them see how things could change and how change was measured. What I really tried to do was to think, shake out my head, and ask myself, "What kinds of things might appeal to the students and be close to their experience so they would not view research as something they took last semester and forgot all about?"

Over the years, as I talked with instructors of research, I tried to help them figure out ways of connecting research to the students' experiences. For example, when evaluating a patient, students are collecting data and evaluating data. The teacher can really tailor the whole course around experiences that students already have so that what is being taught is not something foreign to them. The most important thing I learned over time is that the teacher needs to tailor teaching to the students' experiences. You must start where the students are.

Teaching Dissertation Seminar

At this same time, there were a lot of all but dissertation (ABD) students in the NYU program, and Martha Rogers decided someone should tackle this situation. This was the beginning of teaching the Dissertation Seminar. My job was to gather all the ABD students and help them with their dissertations. I believe that one of the most important things you can learn from situations like this is that you have to begin where people are and that people are pigheaded. I think this is interesting because I too am pigheaded. There is no sense in locking horns with a pigheaded person who really believes they know the situation in which they are entrenched. I find the Socratic method works best and so I begin by asking a lot of questions. Once the person really cannot defend their stance any more, they begin to be open to think differently. Once people start thinking about something else, that sort of breaks up the pigheadedness and they begin to see a little light. Once that happens, they can be a little more relaxed about exploring things that are beyond what they have thought about before. The other thing that I love is confusion. I love it when people are confused, because confused people are learners. People who think they know where they are and what it is all about are not in a position to learn much. Once they get confused, then they want to get themselves unconfused, and it makes for a really ideal learning situation. The teacher needs to be willing to support the student in their confusion even though it may be scary for the student. Once the student gives up a position of being certain, they have to explore and think through unfamiliar areas. I tell students when they say they are confused, "That's terrific! You are beginning to learn and we will get through this, and we always do." There is a lot of information out there about adult learners; teachers have to give them credit for knowing something. They are not beginners. They have been around. Once teachers begin to deal with adult learners, they have to admit that the aggregate of their understanding is way beyond anything the teacher has alone. So, the learning situation can become a two-way street. Both students and teachers are learning together.

FEELING COMFORTABLE AS A TEACHER

After I taught the research course for about 3 years I began to feel comfortable. However, there are a lot of things when it comes to college teaching that go on outside the classroom. Some of this is relating to students with complaints about why you "gave them this" or they "got that." A background in psychiatric nursing helped me immeasurably throughout my whole teaching life and through my administrative career. One of the things I learned was how not to become part of the problem and not to get sucked in by people who are all upset. I am really grateful for my psychiatric nursing background. One thing that is really interesting about nursing students and faculty is that some of them forget the distinction between a patient and a student. Instructors can get entangled by behaving as though students were patients. Patients need to be taken care of, while students are perfectly healthy, normal adults who can stand on their own two feet. One of the things you guide them to do is stand on their own two feet.

CHALLENGES AS A TEACHER

I really wanted to go to the University of Pennsylvania because I knew that I was going to be able to realize many goals as a teacher and as an administrator. However, this meant that I was going to have to move away from home, at least for the week. It took a lot of negotiation with my husband. He was the strangest feminist I ever knew. He was an authoritarian person, authoritarian about everything, and that meant feminism as well. He took the stand that since I deserved this new move I should do it. We negotiated the whole thing. It meant that I had to be away from home, which I was not very happy about. In order to achieve the ends that I hoped for, and be able to realize my own potential, this was the direction I had to take. We both had to come to an understanding about it. It took some hardheaded negotiation, and one of the things that is important in such situations is not to get into, "Yes, but you . . . therefore I . . ." Both are two separate people and what each does has to be considered separately. You are an individual just like the other person is an individual. Ultimately, I believe we all have to give up something to get something.

DEVELOPING POTENTIAL AS A TEACHER

At the University of Pennsylvania I was the Associate Dean for Graduate Studies, teaching Dissertation Seminar, and doing 69 other things. My contact with students was enhanced, not just because of teaching, but also because of where my office was located. I held a philosophy of open doors. I told students and faculty if the chair is empty, then it is yours. During this time, I was able to achieve a closeness to students that I was not able to have before. I think that faculty availability to students is so important, but it is not an issue of "buddy-buddy." Rather, students should feel that they have access to a teacher when they really need it. I have never believed in saying, "Well, let's see, I think I can squeeze you in next Wednesday between 12:00 and 12:30." When people have a problem they want to solve it, and they want to solve it now. My experience is that the longer someone has to wait, the more complicated everything becomes. When I was editing *Nursing Research* and was in the office between 6:00 and 10:00 at night, students got to know I was there late at night and they would say, "The chair's empty, and do you mind?" And actually some of those times, I learned more than what the students learned. I really learned a lot, and believe that these exchanges with students were invaluable to me as a teacher. Having access to students in many different kinds of ways was rewarding. Learning happens outside of the classroom too. For example, when the student tries to avoid taking a course for which the hospital had already paid the tuition, the teacher guides the student to learn that you cannot shrug responsibility. All of these things are part of a learning environment. Penn made it possible for me to create a learning environment that was healthy and sound for students. What goes on in the classroom is just part of the learning. I believe very much in the notion of community in terms of faculty and students together. I think faculty should make learning something that is intrinsically meaningful. People feel attached to their school and are grateful for what they are getting. When I met graduating students, I found that both the students and parents were so proud. All involved had a sense of belonging to something that was important. I do not think any educator can discount the real importance of environment. When I was doing consultation in academic institutions, I could walk into a place and feel what kind of a place this was going to be. I could tell whether the students were satisfied or angry and the impact of the faculty on the students. It was very interesting.

FACILITATING A LEARNING COMMUNITY

In my role as academic administrator I created an environment where both students and faculty had access to the open door and chair. If there were problems, I wanted to know at the time of occurrence so that things could be worked out. I never focus on blame. Things happen and if things did not happen, the administrator would not be needed. I always wanted faculty to tell me what was happening and expected faculty to learn and to teach. I saw myself as the Sheriff. When in trouble, call the Sheriff. The Sheriff will go along with you to take care of things. Not every student can learn. Not every student is in the right place. That's just the way things are. I remember the first student I failed; I felt like a third grade teacher because the student had to take the course over again. I felt just as embarrassed as the student. These things happen. I think it is the ability to have a free exchange, an easy exchange, and without any kind of blame that facilitates solving difficult problems. We had a good time and I loved that job.

EMBARRASSING TEACHING MOMENTS

In that first research course I taught, I prepared the exam and when correcting it found that there was one question that everybody was getting wrong. I wondered how this could be. I went back to my notes, and discovered that I had taught it wrong. At that time, it was called a type-one or type-two error and I had reversed a type-one and a type-two. So I thought, "What am I to do?" Since the class was not going to meet again, I said to myself, "Well, if they ever want to do some research, they can look at their notes and say, gee, I must have taken it down wrong." From that day forward, I taught it as alpha and beta. My attitude is that we all make mistakes. If a teacher makes a mistake, it should not be taken out on a student. In other words, if the student is registered for the wrong course or whatever, the student should not pay because it was not the student's fault that they got in the wrong course. It was the teacher's. I consider it an administrative principle that if one goofs up, say you goofed, move on, and never make the student pay.

REWARDING ASPECTS OF TEACHING

Teaching can be a really fun experience. One of the greatest things any teacher can experience is seeing students grow and become whatever they become. After more than 35 years of teaching, it always makes me feel good when I see students doing great things. It is a terrific reward. Teaching is hard work, and it is also fun. What makes teaching fun and rewarding is that students do learn, grow, and go out and do great things. Teachers have the privilege of seeing them do the great things.

LEAST REWARDING ASPECTS OF TEACHING

I always forget about the least rewarding. There are too many other things that one can worry about.

MAINTAINING EXCELLENCE

I love what I do and am a research buff, a research maven interested in anything about research. I just really like the stuff, and to me it is like being a detective. When I work with someone, what they are doing is trying to see how to make the plan better and cheat the enemy. It is like a game to me. So, it is very hard not to stay good at what you really love doing. To find the solution to a knotty problem is really a lot of fun for me. The question is how to bring the clinical knowledge to bear on the question, so you out-trick the enemy on their own territory. That is such fun. I guess it is a challenge. It's always a challenge. I have had a long, full, and happy life in the various nursing roles I have assumed, and when I hear people complaining about nursing, I do not understand why they wouldn't go and find what would make them happy instead of just going on complaining. There are a million things a person can do.

ADVICE FOR NEW TEACHERS

A new teacher should find somebody who is willing to help them. I think that young faculty members do their best in facing the current high-powered academic environment. It was not easy in the olden days but things are different today. Everything has changed on both sides of the equation. Usually young faculty are teaching undergraduate students in the clinical area and they are expected to publish and to write grants. One new teacher told me that she was expected to secure funding within 2 years. We cannot ask everything from everybody, especially if there is nobody there to help these poor souls. I am working with young faculty and post docs who are trying to get their writing in order. I help them to divide their dissertation in pieces so they can get published and get their priorities straight when they have so much to do. Having someone to talk with about sorting things out and getting organized helps them to do it. For example, I help them in making judgments about whether or not the papers they are writing are for the proper audience and whether they are constructed so they can be understood. These faculty do not have any experience and although they may have a doctorate; it is only the beginning. I believe one of the best things a young faculty member can do is find somebody who is willing to give them a little bit of time, a little bit of a boost, and some direction as to which way to go. I think it would help if more senior faculty realized that someone helped them and that they should take somebody under their wing. That is part of the expectation of an academic community. It is helping people to see that not only did somebody help bring them along, but that everyone has an obligation to the younger faculty as they come in. It is tough to balance and do all this by yourself. Young faculty in nursing are extremely talented; they just need somebody to give them a little boost. There is a need to remember that nursing is not a mature science and that many of the expectations held for faculty in a mature science do not fit. If we insist on making them fit, it would be better not to employ inexperienced faculty in high powered environments.

My view of mentoring is giving people a boost, some direction, and a little help when they need; such assistance is based on a relationship that is akin to a friendship. It is an equitable relationship. A mentor is someone a person feels they can go to, ask questions, and seek advice. They do not have to take the advice. The important thing is to have someone to toss the ball around with, because when people have the chance to talk about things, even if what they came with were the right solutions, they often say, "Thank you for helping me." I often did not help them at all. They helped themselves.

I cannot think of a book that has been helpful to me in developing my expertise in teaching. You know there is no substitute for being an expert in your area, and having some real experience. In the olden days when we were first teaching research, that was the thing we did not have. We were all talking about research and what we knew was our dissertation and that was pretty much it. There was no funding to develop a research career as we now know it. So that when a teacher went into the classroom, you were using examples from the hypothetical, rather than the real. That's one of the reasons why I could teach the whole course in one night.

CHAPTER 5

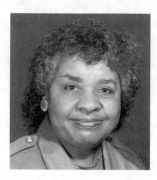

Vernice Ferguson

BACKGROUND

Vernice Ferguson received a BS and Certificate in Nursing from New York University and Bellevue Medical Center, and a master's degree in Health Education from Teacher's College, Columbia University. Ms. Ferguson has held a number of key positions in nursing education and service, including her most recent position as Senior Fellow in the School of Nursing at the University of Pennsylvania, holding the Fagin Family Chair in Cultural Diversity. For most of her career she has been in federal service, as the Chief Nurse at two Veterans Administration medical centers and as Chief of the Nursing Department, Clinical Center, The National Institutes of Health.

She is the recipient of eight honorary doctorates and two fellowships, one in physics, the other in alcohol studies. She is a Fellow in the American Academy of Nursing (AAN); and an Honorary Fellow of the United Kingdom Royal College of Nursing, the second American nurse so honored. She was named a Living Legend of the AAN.

Ms. Ferguson is a past president of the American Academy of Nursing, Sigma Theta Tau International, and the International Society of Nurses in Cancer Care. Ms. Ferguson has published widely in refereed nursing journals and has authored several books including *Educating the 21st Century Nurse: Challenges and Opportunities.*

STORY INTRODUCTION

Vernice Ferguson holds that education is one of the most important issues in nursing. She is a consummate teacher who believes that a vital part of leadership is teaching and mentoring. Her dedication to striving for excellence and the integration of theory and research in nursing is noteworthy.

EARLY INTEREST IN TEACHING

I realized I was interested in teaching during my first assignment as a nurse after graduating from NYU-Bellevue Hospital School of Nursing. I became the head nurse on a funded National Institutes of Health (NIH) research unit, where physicians, physicists, and dieticians who were on the unit taught me. It was my role to guide the nursing staff so that nursing could be a main contributor to the research venture. Thus, I would say in my very first job it became clear that not only did I need to practice as a nurse, but I also had to guide the staff through teaching so that they could do their work.

I am a strong believer in excellence. For me being adequate or mediocre is not good enough in a professional role, you have to be excellent. I entered nursing at a time when women and men were viewed as two separate entities. Men were more powerful than women, and physicians were more powerful than nurses. I thought it important in my career to develop excellence as I grew as a leader. I believed excellence was key to my role in guiding the nursing staff to be their most excellent selves.

PREPARATION FOR TEACHING

I grew up in the era of separate and unequal; the Black world and the White world. In the Black world those who were professionals tended to be teachers, preachers, or physicians. My mother was a public school teacher and my father was a minister who taught many burgeoning seminarians in his study each week. I grew up in a home where every Wednesday night the doorbell would ring, and about six men who were preparing for seminary would go up to my father's study and have class. So, the influence of family roots, including my mother telling us about her early years teaching in a one- or two-room school somewhere in North Carolina was important. In my family, I have two brothers and a sister. Each one has had a teaching assignment at some point in our careers. My older brother was a diplomat, lawyer, and Dean of the Howard University Law School for 10 years during the stormy sixties. He returned to Harvard, where he held an endowed chair in the Law School. My sister was an English literature teacher and taught around the world in Uganda, South Korea, Zambia, and China. My younger brother taught science as I did in the Baltimore public schools. He and I used to have wonderful conversations about what was happening at school. For example, my older brother and I held the view that senior teachers should become engaged as teachers with beginning students. The role models that these teachers become for beginning students are significant. So, I was influenced to teach by my family. Most of my parents' friends were teachers, preachers, or physicians, so that influence has been with me all of the while.

MENTORING FOR TEACHING

I always admired my own teachers in the public schools in Baltimore. We had outstanding teachers. Some were graduates from the Seven Sisters Colleges and Brown University, and because they were Black they were locked into teaching in the public schools. There was nothing else they could do. There were no female broadcasters, or journalists in my era. So, I think my whole upbringing was around people who were teachers, preachers, or physicians, and that became my life. My family mentored me in every way because there were not many Black nurses in our era. My family's friends were my mentors.

My immediate boss mentored me in my first position as the head nurse on a research unit in New York. She and I published together for years after we had been working on problems of calcium metabolism. Her husband, who was the chief of the oncology service, was also a mentor. That physician team of husband and wife were true mentors, and both remained good friends throughout my career.

EVOLUTION AS A TEACHER

In every setting where I worked I inherited traditional nursing services and my role was to turn the situation around. I wanted the people invested in nursing to believe that they could effect change and that I was there to help them with the change process. I believe education changes behavior. So, to me, education is integral to everything I have ever done. My goal was to change behavior so that nurses could be free, more independent, and excited about their work.

For a short time, 4½ years, I left nursing and taught science in the public schools. I taught ninth grade to students in Baltimore, Maryland. During this time, I was fortunate enough to get a National Science Foundation Fellowship in physics. So I had my taste for teaching activated by 4 years in the public schools of Baltimore, Maryland. It was an exciting time. I was assigned to be a supervisory teacher, and did science demonstrations for teachers all over the city. So, even as a beginning teacher, I was teaching other teachers by doing demonstrations.

Then, I taught in a program that prepared licensed practical nurses (LPN) to be registered nurses (RN). Our students had their assignments at Hopkins, and at that time, I was asked if I would join their faculty. I taught Nursing Fundamentals in the diploma program at Johns Hopkins Hospital School of Nursing for about a year. So my beginning formal teaching assignments took place in the public school, in a vocational nursing program, and in a diploma nursing program. All of these came together in the Baltimore area as a formalized teaching engagement. I loved it. However, I was not satisfied to stay exclusively in teaching, I yearned for the challenges of clinical nursing.

Then, the Veterans Administration (VA) recruited me to become a chief nurse trainee. I went to Denver as a Chief Nurse Trainee, and to my first assignment as a chief nurse at the VA Medical Center in Madison, Wisconsin. While there, I had an active teaching assignment. It was teaching oncology at the University of Wisconsin Madison School of Nursing. When I left Madison, I became the Chief Nurse at VA Medical Center in Chicago, Illinois which was across the street from the University of Illinois. There I co-taught the master's seminar with Dean Mary Kelly Mullane. Then, when I came to Washington, DC, I served as Adjunct Professor teaching Nursing Administration and Cultural Diversity at Georgetown University School of Nursing and in the School of Nursing at the University of Maryland. So I consider teaching integral to my career, in each of my Chief Nurse assignments at the VA I maintained an active teaching appointment.

Next, I was invited to join the faculty as Senior Fellow/Fagin Chair for Cultural Diversity at the University of Pennsylvania School of Nursing. While there, we produced two books: *Nursing Education for the 21st Century,* and a *Casebook in Cultural Diversity.* It was a wonderful opportunity to work with faculty from each of the Delaware Valley area schools of nursing. Participating on the team were two nursing faculty from Jefferson, LaSalle, Temple, Villanova, Weidner, Gwynedd-Mercy, and the University of Pennsylvania.

FEELING COMFORTABLE AS A TEACHER

I became comfortable as a teacher when I was successful in my formal teaching experience. I was mentoring beginning teachers. That is when the comfort level set in. It was during my teaching experience in the public school.

CHALLENGES AS A TEACHER

A significant challenge in the public school years was the failure of the schools to have enough equipment for students to learn. I was fortunate to teach in a well-staffed school that had recent textbooks and one microscope for every two students. While across town, my younger brother had old copies of books sent over from the more prosperous schools, and one microscope for 200 students. It was a challenge to have the equipment that you needed to teach in public schools.

However, I did not find that kind of need or challenge when I taught in nursing schools. Whether it was the undergraduate or graduate program, everything that was needed and wanted was in place. The students in nursing were more highly motivated than the public school students. When I taught fundamentals, the students were people who really wanted to succeed in nursing. While teaching the graduate students at the University of Illinois and Georgetown, I found them to be committed to graduate study.

EMBARRASSING TEACHING MOMENTS

I do not recall any embarrassing moments. A funny time that I recall is when I became a public school teacher and took over a class that had seven teachers within 3 months. At this time I was using my married name, which was Vankinscott, and everyone called me "Mrs. Van." I shall never forget when I walked into this ninth grade classroom filled with little hellions and wrote "Mrs. Van" on the board. Then I asked them if they knew what a van does. I told them a van moves things out and if they did not behave and learn science, I would be moving them out. Little did I know the principal was outside the door and he delighted in going downstairs telling the other teachers that if the students did not behave, I was moving them out. That is one funny experience I remember.

REWARDING ASPECTS OF TEACHING

My most rewarding time as a teacher has been the interface with students. It also comes from those students who express how much you have meant to them after the courses are over. Hearing from those I have guided in their work is rewarding. About 2 years ago I received a letter from a former nurse on my staff at NIH who told me she would be retiring from NIH in 108 days.

She wanted me to know how I had helped in her continued growth as a nurse and as a nurse in a research environment. It is those kinds of things that give satisfaction about what I have done. This type of commentary is not uncommon. At Christmastime or at various times during the year, I hear from nurses, from the VA and NIH, who tell me how I helped them to grow and become agents of change.

I encountered a nurse who I did not remember as a student from Georgetown. She is now a nurse attorney in the VA, and shared with me how I had influenced her life. It is that kind of reward that comes after the teaching, rather than while going through it.

LEAST REWARDING ASPECTS OF TEACHING

The least rewarding aspects of teaching are when people fail, cannot get it together, and you must record a failing grade. To me that was always painful because it not only indicated failing on the part of the student, but also failure on part of the teacher because the teacher was not able to reach the student. Failing a student did not happen that often. When it did happen, especially with students who had potential and did not apply themselves, it bothered me. I was concerned that in spite of my best efforts, I could not reach them. That to me is pain. It is not rewarding when students fail to achieve what you believe they are capable of achieving.

MAINTAINING EXCELLENCE AS A TEACHER

One way I maintain excellence is through subject matter expertise. I am an inveterate reader and can never get enough to read. I read the journals in nursing and other health care disciplines. Reading broadens one's mind more than anything else. I try to keep abreast of general trends beyond nursing. Reading keeps me on the edge at maintaining expertise in nursing and beyond nursing. Reading to me is very critical. When I taught the nursing administration graduate course at Georgetown University School of Nursing, one requirement for all students was that they choose an historical or contemporary person and then read that person's biography or autobiography. After reading the book carefully, they were asked to describe why that person was either famous or infamous. This was always a key assignment to get the students in the mode of reading about the lives of people. Whomever they chose, be it Hitler, Alexander the Great, or President

Roosevelt, I wanted to make sure they recognized reading as a way to broaden one's expanse.

ADVICE FOR NEW TEACHERS

I suggest that new teachers find a mentor. The first time in my whole nursing career I felt any sense of a mentor/mentee relationship was with Dr. Mary Kelly Mullane who was the Dean at the University of Illinois School of Nursing. I encourage young teachers to seek out one or more mentors who can help them grow and change. They should seek out people whom they admire. I admired Dr. Mullane. She was a brilliant woman who used language well. The use of language is extremely important to me. For example, a few well chosen words are more important than lots of words. She was a bright lady. So, I would suggest having a mentor.

I would also suggest continuing to grow. One cannot read enough. You can not know all of nursing and health care. The fields are much too broad and constant reading of contemporary literature and seminal pieces in nursing and other health care disciplines is vital.

There is an article written by Rozella Schlotfeldt that appeared in *Nursing Outlook* back in the 1960s, or early 1970s. In this article, she described the nature of nursing and what nursing really is. Not only have I read and reread it, but have also shared it with people who were not nurses so that they would understand the nature of nursing. New teachers need to have a good sense of nursing. It is an embarrassment when professional nurses do not know their roots. You have to keep up, and to keep up you have to keep reading, learning, and studying.

I believe a teacher taps the potential in students by being turned on about what you do. One word sums it all up and that is passion. You have got to have passion. When teachers have a passion about what they do, it gets translated to everyone around them. Teachers should be passionate about their teaching.

Years ago there was a meeting of nurse educators and administrators down in Kentucky, and they asked me to talk about how we prepare our nurse administrators. I wrote an article that appeared in *Hospitals* in August of 1972. In the article, I described my belief that a nurse administrator must also be a teacher. As a nursing administrator I pleaded for a realistic practice and proposed a relevant non-insular educational model for the preparation of future administrators and spoke of the fact that nurses should teach as well as administer, and that researchers should administer as well as teach.

Beyond that I would say it is a world of hard knocks. You just learn by doing, by failing, by picking yourself up, and starting again. It is important for new teachers to be mentored, to have a wide breadth of reading materials, and to be really serious about reading. I can think of no field as versatile as nursing where one has the opportunity all of one's life to teach. Nurses teach other nurses, patients, and other members of the health team. Teaching is embedded in everything a professional nurse does.

In one's career growth, every nurse, however briefly, should actively teach. It is amazing to note the amount of cumulative knowledge that each nurse brings to the day's activities. It is only when it is formalized as a teacher, imparting information to others, that the nurse begins to appreciate the vast storehouse of knowledge that one possesses.

CHAPTER 6

M. Louise Fitzpatrick

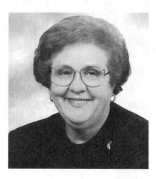

BACKGROUND

M. Louise Fitzpatrick is the Connelly Endowed Dean and Professor of the College of Nursing, Villanova University. She is a graduate of The Johns Hopkins School of Nursing and received a bachelor's degree in nursing from The Catholic University of America. She earned two master's degrees and a doctorate from Teachers College, Columbia University. She holds a certificate from the Institute for Educational Management, Harvard University, is a Fellow of the American Academy of Nursing, and has served as a consultant to numerous schools of nursing and health agencies in the United States and abroad.

Dr. Fitzpatrick has served on the Board of Governors of the National League for Nursing and the American Association of Colleges of Nursing. She is past Chair of the Cabinet on Nursing Education of the American Nurses Association. She has been the recipient of a World Health Organization fellowship for study in Scandinavia and the United Kingdom, and a Malone Travel Fellowship from the Committee on U.S.-Arab Relations. Dr. Fitzpatrick has a strong interest in international health care and nursing education.

STORY INTRODUCTION

Dr. M. Louise Fitzpatrick knew at a very early age that she wanted to be a nursing educator and was mentored by pioneers in nursing education. She holds that teachers of nursing should be grounded in educational theory, academia, and methodology. For her it is most satisfying to have students who have surpassed their teacher.

EARLY INTEREST IN TEACHING

I always thought about being a teacher, even as a child. Also, I used to be a camp counselor and was always around children, so I thought I was going to be a teacher. When I got to high school, for one reason or another, still unclear to me, I became interested in nursing. I used to be a camp counselor for underprivileged children and I could see that there were a lot of health problems that needed to be addressed for these children. Anyway, if you looked at my high school yearbook, every person in that class of 1960 in that small town in New Jersey was asked what they wanted to be. Mine does not say "nurse" and it does not say "teacher." To this day I am baffled by the fact that it says: "Nursing Instructor." I never knew anybody who was a Nursing Instructor, but I guess I figured out that somebody had to teach nursing students.

I applied to a variety of baccalaureate programs but wound up going to the Diploma School at Johns Hopkins because somehow or another a visit there grabbed me. I was an above average, but not an outstanding student for those 3 years of nursing school, until I got to the last experience in community health. It was unusual at that time to have community health in a diploma program and the program at Hopkins was excellent. That is where I really came alive. So, I was out of Hopkins for about one semester working in a New Jersey hospital when I went to Catholic University, and spent 2½ years doing everything that I should have done the first time around to qualify for public health nursing and earn a BSN. It was a valuable experience. Even then, I knew I would become a nurse educator. I went back to New Jersey and did public health nursing for a short period of time and then decided I wanted to go to graduate school. Teaching was still in my mind even though I had not had many years of practice. I was able to gain the practice experience, even as a full-time traineeship supported person because I worked weekends, on call. In addition, during the summers I worked for the Visiting Nurse Service of New York and built up my practice skills. From the very beginning, I knew that I wanted to do something beyond clinical practice and I knew that I did not want to be in a hospital setting.

PREPARATION FOR TEACHING

When I graduated from Hopkins and went home to New Jersey I was practicing as a staff nurse. That following summer, because I had a baccalaureate degree, I was expected to teach the students in that New Jersey diploma school. It was really more clinical supervision than teaching. I did not really know what I was doing, but I knew that I liked the role. Then when I went to Teachers College they had me working with the RNs since I had just finished a master's degree. I taught Community Health Nursing and Maternal Child Health in an outpatient setting. I would have to say that I had some strong influences that moved me to be interested in teaching. One was a music teacher I had throughout my public elementary and high school years. She was a very strong, female role model. My mother was not a teacher, but had gone to law school and graduated in 1929 when not very many women were going to law school. It is interesting that I never had an interest in law. I also had a father who was very supportive of education. I was socialized into higher education at Teachers College, after my initial professional socialization in nursing at Hopkins and my academic orientation at Catholic University. Adelaide Nutting and Isabelle Hampton had been at Hopkins and Nutting then went to Teachers College. I was cognizant of nursing history early on in my career. I cannot identify why or how but I carry that sense of history with me today.

When I entered Teachers College, I was 24 and a full-time student on traineeship. I earned two master's degrees, one in the supervision of public health nursing and one in teaching.

We had some wonderful scholars who were part of our education. Although doctoral study was appealing after I finished my master's I thought I would go out and teach. I had an advisor who was a community health nurse, and she thought that some teaching experience would be useful. In those days when you were young, you listened to what your mentors told you. A conversation took place during which I stood back and heard Frances Frazier and Mildred Montag hold a discussion about me, as if I were not present. Mildred Montag, who was the stronger personality of the two told Fran (my advisor), "I don't care what you say, she is going right on to do the doctorate because this is what other fields do, and our young people in nursing have to do it as well." Then she turned to me and said, "You are going to go right into the doctoral program and I will be the sponsor of your dissertation." However, she added, "You will have to be finished before I retire in 1972," because she said, "I do not plan to carry any doctoral students when I retire." There is nothing like a statement like that to get you moving. Montag's belief was that you demonstrate your research competence through doctoral study and then you move on with your career. She believed that doctoral study was not the capstone of your career, but the beginning of your career. I completed the doctorate in 2 years, 1 week before she retired, and 1 week before I turned 30. I then stayed on at Teachers College in a faculty position. It had been the position of Frances Frazier, my academic advisor, who also retired in 1972.

MENTORING FOR TEACHING ROLE

My faculty colleagues at Teachers College were all very helpful, but I cannot, in all honesty, say that I had just one mentor. Georgie Labadie, although also a new faculty member, had previous teaching experience and became a great friend and helper. She still is a friend today, despite the years and the miles between us. There were my peers like Shaké Ketefian who were not at Teachers College but were sort of going through the same initial experience, and we would get together and talk. The interesting thing was that I was not teaching undergraduate students. I started out teaching graduate students.

Many people influenced me, including a lot of people outside the Department of Nursing Education. The late Professor Walter Sindlinger who was chair of the department of higher education at Teachers College was a wonderful mentor. Even to the day I left and decided to come to Villanova as Dean, Dr. Sindlinger was a wonderful role model. He was a teacher who was knowledgeable in his field, and he understood where the students were, in terms of their education. He was nurturing, supportive, and a good advisor in terms of career development. I would say that he was more of a mentor than the nursing faculty. Eleanor Lambertsen gave me my first opportunity to work as a teacher. Mildred Montag was a very strong personality, the kind of person who motivated you to achieve. She was a Socratic teacher and also played devil's advocate in the classroom. She was never warm and fuzzy, but was very sensitive to the fact that she had young people in the class. She had a sense of history but saw young people as the future. After you sat in her classroom and listened to lectures on curriculum development, you found yourself running to the library to read the dissertation she had mentioned. Before we sat for departmental exams, we had to be well versed in historical documents that were foundational to the development of the field. We were well socialized into what academia was all about. The literature we read went far beyond nursing and nursing education, and

I think that that was very important. We learned what being a professor was all about. I know that some people would probably shudder if they heard me say this, but we were socialized to believe that we were professors and educators first; and our area of expertise or our content area was nursing rather than nurses who happened to be teaching. Therein was the difference. We were expected to be the architects of the educational experience in nursing and assumed the identity of educator.

EVOLUTION AS A TEACHER

I came out of an educational background that socialized women at a young age to a way of thinking that combined the knowledge of pedagogy with expertise in nursing. At Teachers College there was the belief that we should have at our disposal the knowledge and skills to structure curriculum and to understand how people learn and how we should teach to enable learning. We learned to be facile with teaching strategies and the educational principles so that we could assist others who might be clinically competent, but needed help to effectively engage in the educational process. We were educated to be the evaluators, the educators, the curriculum developers, and the educational leaders. It was a rich experience because we took many courses outside of nursing from very accomplished people. Teachers College at Columbia University's School of Education was structured to focus on the history and philosophy of education regardless of one's content area or field.

Courses Taught in Early Career

At Teachers College (TC), I taught all of the Community Health courses including Social and Epidemiological Concepts of Health and Illness. I initially co-taught the course with a colleague, Georgie Labadie, and we were one step ahead of the students. We were not sure what we were doing but in retrospect, I believe that we were teaching nursing theory, which was in its infancy. In addition, I taught courses in long-term care, curriculum development, the practicum for student teachers, and I advised all the nursing history dissertations.

We had huge numbers of students and advisees. The faculty were carrying an unbelievable burden. When I left Teachers College in 1978, I continued to chair the dissertations of 19 doctoral students. All of these students finished within a 2-year period, which was not easy for me as a new Dean living in another state.

In 1978 I went to Villanova as Dean of the College of Nursing. The President was looking for a dean, and my name had been given to him by someone at Middle States. It was at a time when things had become rocky at TC. No matter how hard a few of us tried we could not save the Department of Nursing Education because the administrative support for nursing had eroded. I do not know what made me finally decide to leave. I guess I was frustrated and felt like I could not make a change there. At the time, I was an Associate Professor and in my early thirties. I wanted to be at a place where I thought I could influence something. I never considered going outside of New York and certainly never considered going to Villanova; but the President encouraged me to come and look at the place. He pressed and pressed me and finally I visited in the summer of 1977 but it took until October for me to make up my mind. I said "yes" to Villanova in October. The decision to leave New York was a big one because I'd "grown up" professionally at Teachers College.

I was the only person when I arrived in January 1978 in The College of Nursing with a doctorate. We had a large traditional undergraduate program and I taught the senior trends course. When we started the graduate program 2 years later we began to attract doctorally prepared people to the faculty but they were in short supply. I inherited a faculty that had been there many years. They were an experienced and older faculty, relatively close to retirement who were very supportive of me, even though they knew change was coming. I will always have respect for these women, because they put the school first and themselves second. They wanted the school to grow. They supported what I was recommending and allowed me to make changes and "grow" the faculty. Some people came to us fresh from their master's degrees. I realized that I was not going to recruit doctorally prepared faculty quickly and was going to have to also grow my own. At the present, the faculty consists of 41 full-time persons. About 10 of them were hired as young people with their master's degrees and then went back to school to earn their doctorate. Then I was able to say, "Alright, we will only bring someone in who already has a doctoral degree," which is the case now. So, what I have now is kind of a mixed group of people which includes young PhDs who are ready to roll with their research trajectories, and others whom we grew and are able to participate in the academic process. The hardest thing for me is transforming clinical specialists, or people who are fine clinical experts who decide that they are going to work in the educational environment when they have had no previous contact with that environment. To try and turn them into academicians is a challenge. Clinical specialists come in with a whole different view of the world. They are well

socialized in their role as "nurse" and to turn them into academicians is
sometimes very difficult.

FEELING COMFORTABLE AS A TEACHER

I think it took me about 4 years to really feel comfortable because I was still
quite young (in my thirties), and most of the students that I taught were a
good deal older than I. That alone did not bother me; it was that many of
them were more experienced. I was not intimidated by the students. I can
still remember feeling I had to get through all course content. So I would
say that it took me a good 4 years to really have a comfort level, until I did
not feel that I had to be wedded to the notes in my hands.

CHALLENGES AS A TEACHER

That first course in Social and Epidemiological Concepts of Health and
Illness was a challenge. I had background in Epidemiology, but we were creating a course that was *au courant*. It was very much in line with where the
field of nursing was going but nobody had defined it for us yet. So we were
muddling along trying to do it. It really was a theory course. Georgie
Labadie and I were creating it as we went along.

EMBARRASSING MOMENTS AS A TEACHER

I cannot think of any embarrassing times.

REWARDING ASPECTS OF TEACHING

I think that a teaching career in nursing or a career in educational administration as I am doing now, is probably the most satisfying thing you can
do. I think that if you are a nurse, even though indirectly, you are making
a contribution to health care and to the betterment of mankind. It gives you
great satisfaction to be preparing the next generation to do this work. I
know that in my position now, one of the things I like the most, is becoming involved in larger social issues. I see many opportunities that faculty

may not necessarily identify. Someone may call me and say that there is an opportunity to develop a practice at a clinic for Indonesian immigrants. We can then begin to connect the educational program to some of the needs of communities. This is very satisfying and part of educational leadership in nursing.

Every year we have a career day at our College of Nursing; there is always a panel of alumni in various nursing roles. I said to the faculty, "You invite many alumni back to speak, and they are very interesting, but I do not see one person on that panel who is a nurse educator. There is no one saying, I teach nursing and I think it's a great career." Well, that has changed. They are doing that now. One of my personal missions is to use some of the strategies that our former leaders used in identifying young people and really trying to put them on a career path in which they have interest. I think nursing education is the most satisfying career I could have ever chosen and I want to encourage others to choose it.

The most satisfying experience I ever had and the ones that I most enjoy now are with the international students. I have always been interested in other cultures. At Teachers College we rubbed shoulders with people who were leaders in their fields from other countries. I was always fascinated and made good friends with my international classmates. Then I became a faculty member, and internationals were my students. It was the most satisfying thing to know that you were also making a contribution somewhere else in the world. When I went to Villanova, we were far away from getting involved with international students because we had graduate programs to build. About 12 years ago we were "ready" to have international students and programs and fortunately, the opportunities presented themselves. Now, we have become very international. It satisfies a need in me because I am the happiest with these international students. Patience that I do not have with anybody or anything, I have with this group of students. Our work with the students in the Middle East, especially the graduates of Oman has a 10-year history and I really see a difference in what they are doing when they go back to their country. We feel like we are really making a contribution.

LEAST REWARDING ASPECTS OF TEACHING

I have found my career as an academic very rewarding and cannot think of any parts that are not rewarding.

MAINTAINING EXCELLENCE

Well, I have to be honest with you. I do not do much actual teaching now due to my administrative responsibilities. I will be teaching a curriculum course in the graduate program in the Fall 2004 because someone is on sabbatical. I expect to get more actively involved with the doctoral program. I am excited about that. I think it is very difficult to keep up in your field when you are doing administration. It is a challenge. So, I am not necessarily on the top of my specialty field right now. However, I have stayed conversant with the issues and am an acknowledged leader in nursing and higher education. I think that as new technologies have been made available for teaching and learning that I have really pushed that envelope very hard, so that, technologically we are right where we need to be in our program. One of the things that I try to do, more than anything else, is socialize graduate students and faculty as to what it means to be a professor and what it means to be part of a university.

ADVICE FOR NEW TEACHERS

I would encourage new teachers not to be fearful and to develop confidence. You cannot tell people to be confident; they have to develop confidence themselves. I would try and encourage them to develop a support system. If they do not have the background, e.g., if they do not know how to teach undergraduates, if they do not know how to develop tests, or engage in clinical evaluations they are going to need to learn how to do that. I really feel strongly about it. You know, you just cannot "catch as catch can." In terms of assuming the role, I think that having a support system is important. If they cannot choose a mentor who is more experienced, then they need to create a support system.

It is unfortunate that there is not more exchange among our doctoral students, faculty, and programs. I think that it is sad that the major research universities do not promote this. To socialize a graduate student well is one thing, but cloning them to be like the doctoral faculty is not a good idea, especially in the research universities. What has happened in some instances is that the doctoral mentors clone these students and then, they arrive on the doorsteps of the nursing programs at comprehensive universities or the liberal arts colleges where the primary concern is teaching and they are not prepared for it. And, although part of the agenda is research, they expect more time than can be given, because in most of the institutions where they are employed, undergraduate teaching is still the main enterprise. So, although the major research universities prepare prospective faculty with good research skills, there is something critical that is missing in some of those programs. It seems that as we develop new faculty with strengths in one area, we are losing ground in another, instead of creating a balance. I am all for research, but it is just as important to socialize the students to these other roles of a faculty member. Research should inform teaching and facilitate learning, which is the primary role of the faculty member.

CHAPTER 7

William L. Holzemer

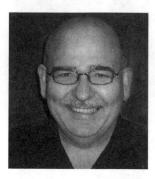

BACKGROUND

William Holzemer is Professor and Associate Dean for International Academic Programs in the Department of Community Health Systems, School of Nursing, University of California, San Francisco. He earned a BS in Psychology from the University of Washington, a BSN from San Francisco State University, an MS in Education/Counseling from Miami University of Ohio, and the PhD in Higher Education Administration from Syracuse University. He teaches a seminar in HIV/AIDS and Adherence and courses in Advanced Quantitative Research Design, Instrument Development, and Measurement of Outcomes.

Dr. Holzemer is a member of the Institute of Medicine, Fellow of the American Academy of Nursing, and a member of the Japan Academy of Nursing. His program of research examines quality of nursing education, quality of nursing care, outcomes research, variation in practice, self-care symptom management, and quality of life, with special emphasis on people living with and affected by HIV infection. He has published more that 100 refereed research articles, edited 6 books, and authored 13 book chapters.

STORY INTRODUCTION

Dr. Holzemer believes that having ongoing feedback and evaluation systems in place with each course is crucial to quality teaching. Even though for the teacher, the assignment is quite clear, the students may find the assignment confusing and become frustrated. He finds the relationships established with doctoral students that extend over time to be a most rewarding aspect of teaching.

EARLY INTEREST IN TEACHING

My early interest in teaching began in early high school. I was a national debater and have always presented in front of audiences. I ran summer camps and taught lifeguard, swimming, and horseback riding. I have been "on the stage" since an early age. I think teaching is a lot like theater; it is a performance. In the beginning, content became what I think of as "tapes you play" in your head. Give me a topic and I will develop a lecture or tape. The importance of content is much more of an issue in the beginning of one's teaching career. Over the years, content has become less important and the engagement and dialogue with the audience has become more important. I have to say though, I never consciously set out to be a teacher. It came with the work.

PREPARATION AS A TEACHER

I entered nursing after earning a PhD in education. Actually, I was planning to go into what one might call student personnel work as an Associate Dean for Students. I was educated in a place where we did extensive work in educational evaluation, along with providing a very good background in research. I had courses in Philosophy of Education, Philosophy of Science, and Futures work. We had training from people out of Illinois, including Michael Scriven, in evaluation. It was an era when evaluation really came into its own as a subdiscipline within education. There was a lot of money at the federal and foundation level to support evaluation work. My first position in nursing was to serve full time as an evaluator of an Advanced Nurse Training grant, designed to prepare faculty for nurse practitioner programs under the direction of V. Ohlson, PD, University of Illinois at Chicago.

I never took a course on how to teach, or how to do overheads, or anything like that.

MENTORING FOR TEACHING

I had a significant mentor for research training, but not to be a teacher. I think I have always had feedback and evaluation systems in place. I believe what mentors a person is discrepancy. If you think things are going well, and all of a sudden you get feedback that they are not, then discrepancy can be powerful in changing how you teach the course. I learned a long time ago that just because it is clear in my mind, it might not be clear with the students. This outlook has mentored me over the years. It can be as simple as an assignment that you think is very clear however; the class is confused about what it is you are asking. Much of my teaching has been in research methods and psychometrics. I always try to give students feedback. Instead of one big term paper due at the end of the course, I give them several small assignments. We have lots of 1- or 2-page assignments instead of one 20–30-page paper. I can remember specifically asking students to mock up what tables might look like for a literature review. They did not understand what I was saying and confusion was created. If things are not really clear, students become frustrated

EVOLUTION AS A TEACHER

I taught for several years a master's research class with 250 students, and that is truly theater. You stand in this hall and you cannot even see the students seated in the back. You learn and evolve over time that you have to be extremely well organized. You do not have the luxury of walking down the hall on the way to class and figuring out what you are going to teach. This type of teaching requires a script, which was a lesson that was hard to learn. In a seminar class you can sort of roll with the process, but you cannot do that in a large lecture-type class.

Some faculty teach by having lots of guest lecturers do their class every week. I have learned over time that this is less effective for me and I do not like this approach. I like to be present interacting and teaching. I do not have many guest speakers. To me it becomes a series of unrelated guest speaker events and does not create an integrated course where the teacher can develop and challenge the students. I think I am of the old school on this approach.

Most of my teaching predates the Web. Today I would have to say that access to content is less of an issue; at least that is what people like to say. However, I believe that part of being a good teacher is providing students with a framework or a road map—which is the vision of where you are going, in addition to required content. I ask a lot of questions, very simple questions. Everyone in the classroom knows what a correlation is. However when you ask them to tell you out loud what it is, a whole different cognitive behavior structure is called forth requiring them to articulate the meaning, as opposed to just knowing silently what it is. Often students are challenged by this strategy. This is one strategy I have used over the years. I push people to go beyond the vague concept of something like an effect size and be able to give me a real, meaningful, concrete example of an effect size.

FEELING COMFORTABLE AS A TEACHER

I still experience being uncomfortable at times. It is like stage fright in a theater. If you have done enough public speaking, you know when things are working and when it is not working. Even today when I know the content through and through and can recite the lecture in my sleep, there are challenges. Who is in the room? What is the environment? What is happening? What happened before? What is happening next? Where they are in their program and training? All make a difference in how things go. You never know if it is going to work or not work. There comes a point when you give a lecture to a large audience where you understand if they are with you or if they are not. This happens to me when I teach. I sense when the group sort of gets on board. I also sense when they are not on board. They may get up and leave, eat their lunch, or let their babies cry. These events happen even when they are with you, but it does not affect you when they are with you. It can all go on if they are engaged.

CHALLENGES AS A TEACHER

I taught the master's level research methods class for about 6 years. There are several classic textbooks that teachers generally use in the course. I let the students choose whatever book they wanted because some of them came to us having purchased these $100 books. The content was mostly the same. I will never forget students standing up and reading to me out of the textbook and saying, "This text said this, but you contradicted the author." Some students were challenged by these disagreements. They really held me accountable and would make me wonder that maybe the book is right. I am quite willing to admit when I make a mistake. These challenges were a lot of fun. I feel uncomfortable when people challenge me at a technical level, yet enjoy exploring the reasons for these apparent contradictions.

When I taught the doctoral research methods courses for 10 years, I became engaged in a mentorship with the students in which many of the relationships lasted from 5 to 25 years. It is not like you are coming in and teaching a course and then going home. You develop friendships and colleagueships that last a lifetime. The workload includes not only teaching the courses but then you move on to qualifying and doctoral committees. A challenge of teaching at an advanced level is that it is not about a course; it is about a career and mentoring people. It is different at a larger master's level course. When you teach a course to over 200 students, people come up to you and say that they have taken your course, and you may not have a clue as to who they are. You simply cannot get to know people when there are 200 in the class. It is a challenge because it is disappointing and sometimes embarrassing.

In the world I live in, we expect everyone to be a good teacher, and what counts is your research productivity. I think the award structure may be changing. When you sit hour after hour reading papers, you think that you could have better spent this weekend writing an article. Reading the same old stuff every year for 10 years gets boring. Teaching the content sometimes gets boring, but working with the students is always rewarding. The technical supports required for a large course is a challenge. For example, you may lose student papers. I always tell students that it is their responsibility to keep copies because I may lose it. One year, I taught the master's research course on Tuesday and Thursday and had trouble remembering what joke that I told or what I had covered. My teaching assistant helped me to remember what I had done in which course.

EMBARRASSING TEACHING MOMENTS

I can't think of any embarrassing moments.

REWARDING ASPECTS OF TEACHING

For the 10 years that I taught the Advanced Quantitative Methods course for doctoral students I was able to stay with them for 20 weeks. It was rewarding to work with students over this extended period of time. Friendships built 20 years ago remain strong today.

LEAST REWARDING ASPECTS OF TEACHING

For 2 years I was involved collaboratively teaching the doctoral course on nursing science. We had four senior faculty teaching it and I thought it was chaos. No one was in charge and everyone was a senior professor. We could not decide who was in charge and who was not. When everyone is in charge, no one is in charge. It was an attempt to bring four very different perspectives into the course. I was systems, another was physiology, another critical care, and another in family nursing. All trying to answer the question, "What is nursing science?" Students hated the course. We quickly changed this course back to having a primary and secondary faculty and the course worked much better.

MAINTAINING EXCELLENCE AS A TEACHER

I have always been a heat seeker. I am always looking out for new technology. I bought the first available desktop computer for $5,000 in 1980 that had a single-sided IBM disk drive. I took a bank loan to buy it and the University thought I was nuts. And so, I started our technology computerization early 1980 and created a lot of opportunities for teaching.

The first 20 years of my life I was viewed as a methodologist. This is how people thought about me and my teaching. Now, because of the work we are doing in HIV care, I do a different kind of teaching. To be competitive in the science, one has to be up on the state of the science in your field. I maintain an active program of research and am fortunate enough to be able to teach in these same areas.

I am launching a whole new area in the New Year as I will be co-teaching the philosophy of science course. That is totally outside my previous areas and I have been retooling myself. I am comfortable teaching philosophy of science from the perspective of clinical trials and NIH and have spent a lot of time reading books and articles to prepare. It makes me nervous because I will be a student learning along with the students in the course.

ADVICE FOR NEW TEACHERS

Teachers in university faculty positions may live in two worlds. First, there is the teaching world of the non-research intensive universities, where teaching is the major area of scholarship. Secondly, there are others, like myself, who work in highly intensive research environments. Quite frankly, teaching can sometimes be a drag on your science. It can hold you back from writing because it takes so much time. I think a new teacher has to first and foremost come to grips with their environment and the concept of scholarship in that environment. Both environments are equally important, however sometimes there is a different reward system. A 4-year private college that has a nursing program where scholarship is at the interface of teaching, community service, and practice is one world. However, if you are in a major research intensive university, I think you have to protect your time carefully. One of the biggest problems is over-teaching. I advise new faculty in research intensive environments to be very astute, to select their courses carefully, and stay with them for at least a 5-year cycle. The "kiss of death" for a beginning scientist is to change your teaching assignment every year or every term to teach a new course. These are issues of control over one's environment that I think are very important. New teachers should negotiate the areas in which they will be the expert teacher, develop these areas over time, and by all means stay with them. New faculty should resist in being jerked to teaching community one year, pediatrics another, and then research methods the next year. Focus, focus, focus.

There is a whole arena of scholarship in teaching that I spent 10 years trying to develop at the National League for Nursing and starting The Society for Research in Nursing Education. We published six annual reviews of nursing research. Research funds moved away from nursing education to patient-focused clinical research. However, there remain tremendous challenges in the scholarship of teaching, interdisciplinary teaching, and multidisciplinary teaching.

Another piece of advice for new faculty is to remember that, every time you want to change the curriculum, drop the idea and get on with your science. Nursing has a real demand and a real challenge to keep their curriculum linked to practice and the demanding clinical environment. At the same time, massaging the curriculum ad nauseum is one of the greatest excuses for not publishing and not doing research. I would very judicially and very carefully pick the time when curriculum needs to be changed. Try to resist it at all costs because it will never be perfect and it is constantly in need of changing. The curriculum has to have some degree of freedom to flex. The challenge is to build the knowledge base through the natural and human sciences that will inform evidence-based practice. Good teachers build and disseminate this evidence.

I encourage new faculty to work with doctoral students if you have the opportunity. These students become friends and colleagues. I have always believed that mentoring is a mutual process, and it regenerates you as a faculty person. Work with people who have different backgrounds than your own. Have fun because I believe our work is about the journey, not the destination. Become the students' coach and facilitator. The teacher is not the person who has the most knowledge, rather the one who facilitates and supports the learner. This requires a different comfort level because it is more demanding and it requires your engagement. Technologies for teachers today are not an option. It is a requirement and you have to figure out how you will interface with the technology.

I started my career working collaboratively in medical education in 1975. Schools of medicine usually have departments of medical education, recognizing that medical faculty may not have expertise in teaching and evaluation. Schools of medicine have enough resources to have a department of medical education, which helps them build their examinations, their clinical simulations, and their curriculum. Nurses for many years were educated in schools of education so they had these skills. This is not true today. New faculty are encouraged to work in settings that provide support for our teaching, in areas such as technology, curriculum development, and testing and evaluation. Developing expertise as a teacher-scientist is a challenge. My advice is to create a nurturing environment for yourself so that you can provide such an environment for your students.

CHAPTER 8

Pamela Ironside

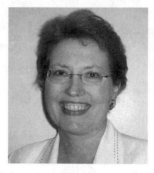

BACKGROUND

Pamela Ironside is an Assistant Professor of Nursing at the University of Wisconsin-Madison. She earned a BA in nursing from Luther College, an MSN from the University of Minnesota, and the PhD from the University of Wisconsin-Madison. She teaches a variety of nursing education courses including curriculum development, instruction, and clinical education.

Dr. Ironside's current research uses interpretive phenomenology to explicate how new pedagogy influences thinking in classroom and clinical courses, reforming practices in nursing faculty, and the experiences of nursing doctoral students. She is a member of the Board of Governors of the National League for Nursing (NLN) and served as an invited member of the NLN's think tanks on graduate preparation for the Nurse Educator Role and on Standards for Nursing Education. She was recently appointed as a site evaluator for the Commission of Collegiate Nursing Education. She is associate editor of the book series, *Interpretive Studies in Healthcare and Human Sciences* and is the editor for Volume IV, titled *Beyond Method: Philosophical Conversations in Healthcare Research and Scholarship*. In addition, her work is widely published in health care and nursing journals.

STORY INTRODUCTION

Dr. Pamela Ironside moved to nursing education after rising through the ranks of nursing administration. She believes in a nonstructured approach to the teaching/learning session and likes to begin class involving students in discussion of questions, thus inspiring a spirit of inquiry. She views students as partners in learning.

EARLY INTEREST IN TEACHING

I have always been interested in teaching. When I graduated with my baccalaureate degree, I worked in a surgical trauma/intensive care unit. I was often asked to work with students who would come to the unit for an observation experience. Even though these experiences were for observation, I tried to explain everything that was going on and to help them make links between what they were seeing and what they were learning in their program. I found that this felt like a natural thing to do and I found I looked forward to these experiences. Then I took the position of Assistant Head Nurse and in that position I was in charge of staff development and orientation. This experience was delightful. I found teaching was the part of my job that I really liked, in part because it kept me learning new things. After rising through the ranks of administration, I found that I missed teaching. When my family decided to relocate, we decided to move to a place we wanted to live rather than to a job. So we relocated to Minnesota and there happened to be a position open at the College of St. Scholastica (CSS) School of Nursing.

PREPARATION FOR TEACHING

At first I was not prepared, my master's degree was in nursing administration. I was very fortunate that the school I was teaching at was very good. I was able to spend an entire quarter with the faculty, watch them teach, and talk with them about teaching. They were very generous with their time and ideas as I planned for my first course. So, it was not as if I had no preparation, but the preparation was not formal preparation. At CSS, they provided courses that were interdisciplinary for all new faculty on writing exams. There were a series of four each year. That got me started in developing skills in teaching. It was not until I went back for my doctorate that I decided I wanted to do more in nursing education. Even though I think I did OK in my role at CSS, I knew there was so much more that I didn't know. I really wanted a background in education, to do research in education, and to learn about research and design issues so I could make a difference to nursing students and teachers. I earned my doctorate at the University of Wisconsin-Madison. It was in my doctoral experience that I really focused on learning about nursing education.

MENTORING FOR TEACHING

When I came to work with Nancy Diekelmann, I had taught for 3 years. Her work in using Heideggerian hermeneutics to study nursing education really engaged me in thinking about teaching and learning in a new way. At first, I observed and taught along with her. I would respond to various situations and we would talk about what was going on. I started teaching graduate courses using Narrative Pedagogy, even though I had never taught that way before. We would talk about my concerns, how the class might go, what kinds of questions might come up, and things that I needed to think about. We never talked about content issues. This was very helpful to me. The most important thing to me about her mentoring me as a teacher was that she had undying faith in me—she persistently communicated her belief that I could do it. She never once was harsh, condescending, or critical. She was always positive with specific examples of what might work in a given situation. She instilled in me the spirit of inquiry—encouraging me to try new things or ideas, see what happens, and then we would talk about what worked and what didn't. This is something that I try to instill in every student I work with. Still after all these years, I can watch her teach and learn something new about how she engages with students and gets them thinking together about new possibilities for teaching and/or research.

EVOLUTION AS A TEACHER

When I first began teaching, I was teaching as I had been taught. I constructed lectures and had every aspect of the class preplanned. I was very clear about where I would be at any time throughout the lectures. When I was really new at teaching, I would time the lectures and practice them at home. I would put little sticky notes on my lecture notes so I could monitor where I was related to what I had planned. As I became more comfortable, I "let go" of my notes a little more. Then I realized how much more interesting the class became and how much more engaged the students were when I would start talking about my own experiences in caring for patients in different situations. This approach started creeping in more and more into the class. It took me a while to get confident enough that I knew what I was talking about to begin relying more on discussion and engaging students' thinking. I soon began to realize how I had a lot to offer and that the students had a lot to offer too. I began to worry less about whether or not I could not answer every question. Then I was able to try more new things and really follow the students' questions and concerns. I tell new teachers now that when you are most unfamiliar with the content, you really want to hang on to control in the class. Now I like to start out the class with questions that I have and do not know the answers. I bring my questions to class and have students investigate them. This approach has been really helpful. At this time, my classes are nonstructured. I deal a lot with drawing from the students' experiences and questions and we collectively work on interpreting and re-interpreting these experiences throughout the course. It is more meaningful and engaging for me and I think for the students as well.

FEELING COMFORTABLE AS A TEACHER

My feeling comfortable is best described on two levels. After the first couple of years I was comfortable enough that I could teach a course well. Yet, with every new class, I am never really comfortable even when it is a course I have taught many times. There is always both excitement and worry with every new class. I work very hard to stay mindful because I want to hold on to how difficult it is for students to learn. I often reflect on my own experiences as a student. I think I am a better teacher when I keep myself learning something new and remember how overwhelming learning can be. Therefore I am always a little uncomfortable. This experience helps me appreciate how hard students are working.

CHALLENGES AS A TEACHER

Probably the biggest challenge is in clinical instruction that involves being moved to units that are not in your area of expertise. When schools were trying to secure clinical sites, we had to move to wherever the sites were located. I worked hard as a teacher to help students learn new skills and how to think in rapidly evolving situations. I was worried about the patients, and what I was not picking up on, because I did not know the specialty like I knew other specialties. That has been a significant challenge that clinical teachers continue to face.

EMBARRASSING TEACHING MOMENTS

I was using an overhead projector when teaching my first large lecture class, and for whatever reason, I always had it backwards so that it projected the image on the ceiling. In the end-of-year celebration at this school the students did skits. They came in and projected the overhead on the ceiling, and said, "What teacher is this?" It has kind of followed me around. Every once in a while, students will make you aware of your little mannerisms that you do not know you are showing in class. Another thing was in one of my nursing education courses I taught where we were talking about student evaluations of faculty. The students were master's students so they had been students for a long time. They did not believe that faculty ever really saw what they wrote on their evaluations. So the entire class wrote on their evaluation, "I wish she was taller." Sure enough, the student comments report came back with 10 identical comments, "I wish she was taller!"

REWARDING ASPECTS OF TEACHING

I am rewarded when I see teachers teach in ways that are more student-centered and that create warm, receptive environments for learning nursing. I am also rewarded when I see students thinking in ways that challenge underlying assumptions and create new possibilities. I like seeing students develop confidence in their intellectual abilities and to begin seeing themselves as nursing scholars.

LEAST REWARDING ASPECTS OF TEACHING

It is least rewarding when arguments persist about the curriculum and what content goes where. Too often, at the end of the day, it is really not different in any substantive way. This creates tensions among faculty and takes an incredible amount of time and energy.

MAINTAINING EXCELLENCE AS A TEACHER

I try hard to listen very well to students. Students will really help you out about what is a good idea, what is not working, and what you can do to fix it. When I was a new teacher, it was easy to become defensive with students and to spend time trying to explain all the reasons why I was doing what I was doing. But I've learned that when you listen to students, really listen to them, they will not let you down. They just make you a better and better teacher and they help you make your courses more and more compelling. I also try to take continuing education classes and put myself in situations where I am a learner. I do a lot of reading and try a lot of new things in my courses. I'm lucky to be able to do research in teaching and learning because what I learn in my research helps me be a better teacher.

ADVICE FOR NEW TEACHERS

The best advice I could give is to see students as your partners in learning. Pay attention to how they are experiencing your course, and listen to what they have to say. Do every assignment you ask students to do. You will gain a lot of insight into which ones work well and which ones don't, and which ones are compelling and which are either too difficult or are busywork. Talk to students a lot. I really believe that students will not let you down. They will step up and go beyond your expectations and be creative. If you have a really good idea, try it. And last, but not least, I would stress the importance of research in nursing education. If we want an inclusive science of nursing education to guide our teaching practice we must all get involved in making that happen.

CHAPTER 9

Pamela R. Jeffries

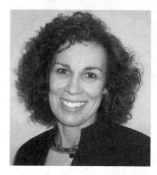

BACKGROUND

Pamela Jeffries is an Assistant Professor of Nursing in the Department of Adult Health at the Indiana University School of Nursing. She earned the BSN at Ball State University, and the MSN and DSN at Indiana University. She has over 20 years teaching experience in the classroom, learning laboratory, and clinical settings with undergraduate nursing students. She also facilitates Web-based courses in critical care and a graduate level course on teaching in nursing.

Dr. Jeffries is Project Director of a multisite research project aimed at studying various parameters related to the use of simulation in basic nursing education programs and selected student outcomes. Her research and scholarship of teaching are focused on studying learning outcomes, instructional design, new pedagogy, innovative teaching strategies, and delivery of content using simulated learning. She is published widely in books and journals.

STORY BACKGROUND

Dr. Jeffries loves her work. She finds every day exciting and is never bored. She has moved from a teacher-centered approach to education to a student-centered approach. She balances her family life with her role as an educator and she lets students know her background and educational experience up front so that students have an opportunity to see her as human. She believes that her expertise as a teacher has been shaped by strong relationships with her mentors.

EARLY INTEREST IN TEACHING

I always wanted to be a nurse and decided during my senior year in high school to attend nursing school. My first work experiences were in surgical and critical care nursing, and I seemed to be always the nurse orienting and precepting graduate and other staff nurses. At the time, I think of those activities as teaching, but I always assumed the mentoring role in trying to guide others. Others would seek me for mentoring, but also I would volunteer. Then in 1982, I was working on my master's and also working in critical care, with a lot of overtime. I heard that a part-time teaching position was available in cardiovascular nursing at a nearby university. Since I was working in a critical care unit at that time I thought it might be a good fit. The part-time position ended up being full time and I never turned back. I loved it. I was very busy, but very engaged.

PREPARATION FOR TEACHING

During the early 1980s, while I was working on my master's degree, I took some teacher education courses taught by Dr. Freda Scales. She was wonderful and I learned a lot from her; that enticed me more. That was my formal education for teaching for my master's degree, two courses in teacher education. In my doctoral program my major was nursing synthesis and my minor was higher education. As electives for my minor in higher education, I had several education courses, including courses in instructional design. That was before I knew I was going to focus on multimedia, CD-ROM, and on-line educational development. I also took general courses in higher education, but I did not have any nursing education courses in my doctoral program. The doctoral program at Indiana University (IU) was very rigorous in research. To prepare myself as a teacher, I was like a sponge to any education materials to help prepare me to be a better clinical instructor. I read all kinds of literature, including self-help books and journals.

MENTORING FOR TEACHING

In the early 1980s, when I started teaching, I encountered my first mentor; her name was Anitta Hamilton. She hired me for my first teaching position and was course leader for the cardiovascular module that I taught. She was a super lady—very organized and a very good educator. She peer reviewed my teaching and my grading. I was a first-time educator and felt that I received important mentoring from her regarding my teaching. If I was too harsh in grading, or not harsh enough, she would give me constructive feedback. I never felt criticized, just supported. Once I got my doctorate, I was hired as an assistant professor at IU in the tenure track and assigned a mentor, Dr. Diane Billings. She has been my mentor since then, and the world knows it, not only in teaching, but also for research and for overall scholarship. As a junior faculty member, I felt supported not only by Dr. Billings, but by the system at IU and also by my Dean, Dr. Angela McBride. They have helped mold me.

EVOLUTION AS A TEACHER

Back in the 1980s when I first started, teaching was very teacher-centered, with students in a passive role. I was trying to get a 3-hour lecture in with heavy medical surgical content. Then in higher education there was the paradigm shift from teacher-centered to student-centered teaching and learning. I wanted to do that, as I saw the positive outcomes of student-centered learning. During my pre-doctoral and doctoral teaching experience I was very much teacher-centered. When I entered the tenure track position at IU I became more student-centered in my teaching. One of the areas for my teaching was the learning lab. Dr. Juanita Laidig was the undergraduate curriculum coordinator at the time. She had a strong influence on me and my teaching. She told me our learning laboratory methods needed to be upgraded; at that time they were organized for very passive learning. As the learning lab instructor I had five students for 2 hours of lab. The model was that we would lecture to them for the first hour and by the end I was falling asleep and they were falling asleep. Then I would demonstrate the skill to the students and there might or might not be time for them to practice. Usually the lab time was focused on one skill set. With support from Dr. Laidig, I changed the laboratory to become student-centered with students taking responsibility for their learning through participation in interactive modules. We even had lab kits that they could take home to practice their skills and they could check out CD-ROMs and videos. My teaching role shifted and I became a facilitator of learning. No longer was I providing all of the information for students; I held them accountable for their own learning through self-study modules. We set up six interactive labs and over a 3-week period the student would rotate through the labs. They could build on their experiences, and many of the students did so. They could spend more time on the skills for which they needed more practice. There was a lot of skepticism expressed by other faculty because the students seemed to be moving all over, had too much energy, and were talking all at the same time. My skills lab was not in a small defined area where I had control. We had 50 students rotating through six different stations. Fortunately, we had a parallel curriculum that was being phased out, and this provided an opportunity for me to do a study comparing the two teaching-learning methods. I had two doctoral students evaluate the course assessing two different types of learning outcomes. The learning outcomes for the student-centered versus the teacher-centered lab were similar, but the students were more satisfied with the student-centered approach. Now when I go to a committee meeting and I hear support for student-centered learning I am pleased that I conducted and published that early study.

Another area in which my teaching has evolved over time is related to the platform from which we teach. Right now, I am teaching two on-line courses, one graduate and one undergraduate, and have students from all over the United States. In the undergraduate course, which is focused on critical care, we have a triad of participants: myself as a teacher, the student, and the clinical preceptor.

FEELING COMFORTABLE AS A TEACHER

I do not remember ever feeling uncomfortable as a teacher. I remember my first lecture was on the heart; I was an expert clinician in cardiac care and the senior level nursing instructor and felt very comfortable with that content. My course leader was there with me, observing from the back of the room. She was doing peer review, but I knew she was there to be helpful. I knew the material and I was not uncomfortable. The hardest part was worrying whether I had enough content for the 2-hour lecture. I think my clinical expertise and the support I felt from my colleagues made me feel comfortable in my teaching. My teaching evaluations were always good, and that increased my confidence. Though I have had different types of students—associate degree, BSN, graduate, clinical, laboratory, didactic, large classrooms, small classrooms—I have never felt uncomfortable, even in clinical teaching. I remember taking 12 students at once to clinical rotations and many times I taught them fundamentals, yet I never felt uncomfortable. I did always feel challenged to make sure that the students were not making errors. I delineated the guidelines and made sure they were accountable for preparation for the clinical experiences. The students always knew my expectations.

CHALLENGES AS A TEACHER

I always felt challenged as an educator to prepare a good lecture, a creative lecture. I wanted to be innovative. I did not want to do a 3-hour talk just to talk. That was before changing my focus to experiential learning and interactive activities. I tried to make learning enticing. I wanted to use good overheads. I always felt that as an educator I wanted to display professionalism, in the way I talked, acted, dressed. I did not consider myself the students' role model because I think the clinical nurses should be their models, but I still wanted to display professionalism. The challenge was always to prepare good lectures and good clinical experience for students. Other challenges were challenging students themselves, including some of those who were at the lower level of performance. I vividly remember two students who presented challenges; one who lied and did not have integrity; I was appalled. I could not imagine someone in nursing school without personal integrity. She was dishonest about such things as saying she did a dressing change when she did not and other treatments that she claimed doing. Another challenging student was one who was lacking in the basic knowledge and skills to be a nurse. I had to fail both of these students, but both of them understood.

EMBARRASSING TEACHING MOMENTS

Embarrassing teaching experiences include the student who was giving her first IM injection. This is a big hurdle for most students, so any time we performed this skill, we would rehearse it first. Then we would go into the patient's room and the student would do the intervention. I was there with them, but tried not to interfere unless there was an unsafe behavior. So this student was ready to give the injection and got into position, and then she jumped on the bed to get a better grasp for the injection. She was literally in the bed, almost lying right next to the patient trying to get the right angle!

One time, a staff nurse told me one of my students had taken her coffee into the patient's room and was drinking her coffee at the bedside, with the patient who was comatose. Another funny moment was in the learning lab, where I had set up an assessment for a structured clinical evaluation. I had used a real person simulating a patient at a station where a student had to hang an IV piggyback on a fake arm. The student was supposed to ask him if he had any allergies, but the real patient was conversing with the student as she hung the piggyback. The student came out of the cubicle crying and extremely upset that she did not finish that station. She said, "I was hanging this piggyback and my patient was talking to me!" I said, "Yes. They do that." I was totally caught off guard that she was so alarmed. That made me realize that we needed to provide more realistic experiences for our students.

REWARDING ASPECTS OF TEACHING

The most rewarding aspect of teaching is helping students achieve their goals. I remember in a didactic course a student had to get an 82% on one test in order to pass the course. She had never gotten that high a score before in this course. I worked with her and she got an 88%. Another reward has been the recognition I have received from students as an outstanding faculty member. This recognition is not political but rather it is the students, from their hearts, acknowledging you. Also, rewarding for me is the development and testing of instructional multimedia with students such as those who I have taught on-line. It is rewarding to hear them say, "Wow, this is great! I can learn from this. I like the organization. I love all the videos. I can rewind the video and replay how to give medications." Putting those products out there and developing them with the students in mind is so rewarding to me. Another reward is having my peers recognize me for my teaching. I have received all-university and departmental teaching awards; having my peers recognize me for my teaching is very rewarding because you never really know what your peers think, until something like that occurs.

Another reward was when I was in a school nurse role, in an international school in Indonesia where there were 210 children, preschool through grade 10, and an eclectic curriculum with 26 different cultures represented; this was an awesome experience. I became a health educator and I developed a health and personal development curriculum. These young children did not know about drugs and alcohol or tobacco. They did not know about healthy decision making. I incorporated all of this in my teaching as a school nurse. Mind you, as a "razzmatazz" American, coming and doing a drug awareness program, the parents were wondering, "Who is she?" I had morning coffees with these parents from different cultures, explaining that I was stating the facts and promoting healthy decision making. I had to make it clear that I was not telling their children to engage in these behaviors. To educate these children, and at the same time, their parents, was so rewarding. We had a drug awareness program and students came back after the summer and thanked me for providing them with knowledge. During this time I also taught many people CPR; that was so rewarding since these were important skills the expatriates may have to use sometime in their lives.

LEAST REWARDING ASPECTS OF TEACHING

It is hard to think of negative aspects of teaching because I always like what I do. I am more optimistic and positive than not; I try to find the good in what I do, even in developing new projects or programs. Going through development is somewhat less rewarding, e.g., curriculum revision. At one time I was responsible for 2–3 courses in the undergraduate program that required major revamping of the curriculum. I felt overloaded when doing this since even with my background in multimedia I was not sure whether I was developing the courses appropriately.

MAINTAINING EXCELLENCE AS A TEACHER

To keep up, I read all the time, including new journals and about new innovations. I attend conferences, like the NLN Summit directed toward nurse educators. I continue to have peer reviews and am an elected member of our university's faculty teaching colloquium. This group includes outstanding faculty from the entire university, not just from nursing. They hold retreats and I feel uplifted. I attend workshops on on-line development, Web design, and so forth in order to learn different teaching strategies.

ADVICE FOR NEW TEACHERS

My advice to new teachers is to be yourself. One of the most important things that students need to know is that teachers are human. We are just like them. We have a job to do. At the beginning of every course I have, whether for 100 students, 30 students, or 10 in my clinical group, I talk about my professional background and experience and what I bring to the table; I also bring up my 4 children. They know I am a mother; they know I am balancing family life with my role as a teacher. I am an educator but I also have a personal life.

If I make a mistake, I want the student to tell me. I listen to students. I even have students coming back after they leave my class because they think I am a good listener. Sometimes, as a teacher, I can decrease students' stress by altering their deadlines. For example, on my on-line courses, I had a student working on the weekend. I happened to be on-line on Sunday. She was on-line posting that she was trying to get the attachment. I could sense her frustration, even on-line. I posted, "Call me now." She called within 10 minutes, and we worked it out. I say to new teachers, whatever you do, continue to evaluate your own behavior. I do not go in with the notion that what I do is perfect, or that it is going to work. Until you evaluate yourself, you do not know. I do not assume that I am doing everything right, and I do not assume that the students know the answers to even the most simple or obvious questions. Treat the students as you want to be treated. I model my teaching after the way I was treated by the good teachers I have had in my own learning experiences. I try to understand their predicament. When the students do poorly on a test, I do not automatically assume they did not read or study. I look at my teaching and think that I did not get that concept across. I love my job. Every day is exciting to me and I am never bored. I always have many projects going at once. I get excited about education, I really do not understand why more people do not come into education. The scholarship of teaching and learning is so important. Look at best practices in education. Look at the literature. Contribute to the literature. Conduct research in nursing education. Nursing research is not all just about clinical outcomes and clinical research, but also includes educational research.

CHAPTER 10

Patricia R. Liehr

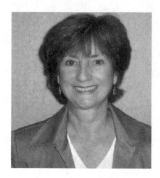

BACKGROUND

Patricia Liehr earned the BSN from Villa Maria College, MSN from Duquesne University, and PhD from the University of Maryland. She also completed a postdoctoral program at the University of Pennsylvania in Clinical Nursing Research. She is Professor and Associate Dean for Nursing Scholarship at Florida Atlantic University, Christine E. Lynn College of Nursing. She began studying story with her dissertation, where she examined blood pressure changes while talking about a normal day and while listening to a story. The connection between story theory and bodily experience continues to be a thread in her research. She and a colleague have created a middle range theory of story proposing that story is a narrative happening of connecting with self-in-relation through intentional dialogue to create ease. Dr. Liehr believes that stories are powerful entities for not only chronicling but also creating health.

STORY INTRODUCTION

Dr. Liehr was not prepared and not even mentored when she began her early career in teaching. She remembers it as being scary. She was helped along the way by good teachers who modeled Socratic questioning and engaged students actively in the process of learning. As she has matured, she experiences herself becoming more comfortable and grounded in her teaching. Her intent when with students is to be open, encouraging, and present while always ready to hear and listen. She keeps her teaching vibrant and her scholarship up to date by not taking on activities that pull her away from teaching and scholarship. Another way she keeps focus is "weeding her committee-work garden" every 6 months.

EARLY INTEREST IN TEACHING

The first time I thought about moving from practice to teaching was before I finished my baccalaureate degree. I graduated from a diploma program and then went on to earn a baccalaureate degree. While I was in the process of completing the degree, I had been working in critical care. At this particular time, I was working at St. Vincent's Hospital in Erie, Pennsylvania, which had a 3-year school of nursing. It was a Catholic institution and one of the nuns at the School of Nursing asked me if I was interested in a teaching position. I was flattered that she asked me and viewed it as an exciting possibility. I applied and was hired to teach. This was the first time I ever thought about teaching.

PREPARATION FOR TEACHING

I was not prepared, and I was not even mentored. I had not yet earned my baccalaureate degree, and there I was teaching. I remember having hives because I was so nervous about not knowing what to say to the students. I remember sitting in the faculty lounge with hives. As much as I wanted to do it, it was scary.

My next position in teaching was in the baccalaureate program, after just having received my own baccalaureate degree. This was at Slippery Rock State College. Slippery Rock had just started their baccalaureate program and they were desperate for faculty. So at this point I enrolled in a master's program. It was as if the teaching positions drove my education. Actually, it was the need for teachers that drove my education. I do not recall anyone ever helping me with my teaching, as far as how to do it. I was on my own. Then in the baccalaureate program, I recall there were faculty who were supportive. However, there was no structured way of helping me.

MENTORING FOR TEACHING

What helped me was having good teachers in my master's program. At that point, I was a student in Duquesne University's master's program in nursing and there were senior expert teachers. I have always thought that my education there was one of the best experiences I have ever had. I watched how the faculty asked questions, in a Socratic sort of method. This opened a new way of being in a classroom for me. I did not know how to do this sort of questioning but I liked the way the questioning engaged the student so I started doing that with my students. Because I had no education about how to teach, I figured things out myself. For example, when I had to put a syllabus together, I would find a copy of another syllabus and see what went into the syllabus. I never felt confident about tests because I was not confident about my questions. Students could almost always argue me out of "the correct" response because they would make another rationale for my questions and I could see their perspective.

EVOLUTION AS A TEACHER

I believe I have evolved through my personal growth. Over time, as I have become more mature and more comfortable with who I am, I have become more grounded in my teaching. I do not feel like I must have a right answer every time. I see students as my teachers. I do not see myself as the teacher. I am engaged in a dialogue with students and we are both learning at different levels. Therefore, I try to maximize the dialogue. To do this takes a personal maturity and it does not happen quickly. Engaging the students in dialogue is really about story. It is also about being open to where the student is and not feeling threatened. Even when I feel uncomfortable, I try to hear what they say, even if it sounds like a real challenge, or disagreement, or even an insult. I try to move away enough from the emotion to come back and explore where that student is in a way that is enlightening for me, and usually enlightening for the student. In my mind it is the intention to listen and to hear. Therefore my intent is to be open and to encourage understanding. If I approach a student with this intent, and the student does not grow in understanding, then I cannot help that. However, my intent is to always be present to the student.

FEELING COMFORTABLE AS A TEACHER

When I began teaching at Duquesne University, I still was not comfortable. I was in my master's courses at Duquesne and was teaching undergraduate classes, part time, while I was getting my master's. I was not comfortable because I was still growing who I was in nursing. Then, I went into the doctoral program and was teaching graduate statistics at the University of Maryland. I still was not comfortable. Then there was an interlude where I did postdoctoral work and did no formal teaching. After postdoctoral work, I went to the University of Texas and after a couple of years I began feeling comfortable. I was there for 15 years. I believe it is as much about age and maturity as anything.

CHALLENGES AS A TEACHER

Balancing time by keeping my teaching alive and vibrant and my scholarship up to date is a challenge. It is an additional challenge when practice and administrative responsibilities are added. The challenge is to find a balance. The challenge is bigger than just teaching. It is putting it all together. It has always been my view that I am not a teacher, I am a nurse. My primary way of being is as nurse and researcher. I teach to express what I know as nurse and researcher. I have never viewed myself as a teacher. However, I recognize that I have a responsibility to the people who are coming after me. I have been blessed to be able to earn a doctorate and to do research. It is my responsibility to share what I learn in these ways with students. One of the ways I keep the balance, because students always demand time, is to block out time for scholarship. I keep one day a week for scholarship. It is important that my research grows and develops so that I can continue to share meaningful ideas with students. I work to not keep pushing scholarship aside. It is critical to stay with the scholarship.

Now, since I have recently moved, I am considering how I can contribute to the mission of the College as the Associate Dean of Nursing Scholarship and keep my scholarship alive. I try not to take on things that are going to pull me away from my direction. For example, I generally try to work with doctoral students who are interested in story. I try to keep a focus, even in my teaching. When I mentor a student to submit an NRSA (National Research Service Award), and the NRSA uses story method, the time spent on the NRSA pulls the teaching and research together. Another way I have kept my focus is to "weed my committee-work garden" every 6 months. I look at all the things I am doing, committee-wise, and think which ones are most important and which I can stop.

EMBARRASSING TEACHING MOMENTS

There was an embarrassing time with the Thai students in dissertation seminar last year. There were three Thai students, and several American doctoral students who I was mentoring. In one of the dissertation seminar classes, the Thai students brought in ears of corn. Every now and then a student would bring in something for us to munch on because these classes went from 4–7 in the evening. It was an informal seminar. After looking at these ears of corn, I looked around and sort of shrugged at this unusual treat. I thought since the Thai students had brought it I had better eat it to show respect for the gift. I picked up my corn and ate it all off and the other teacher present in the group ate it all off too. Then, what I noticed about midway through the class was that no one else had eaten any corn. I then noticed one of the Thai students taking off the kernels of corn one by one. She was eating them one at a time, taking one, eating it, taking another and eating it. The students were discussing their research but I said to the Thai student, "You eat the corn very differently." She softly said, "One by one." All of the students learned a lesson about cultural dimensions of social interaction as we discussed how the other teacher and I ate the corn. I believe the point of this story is that you sometimes learn what you least expect to learn in a teaching situation.

REWARDING ASPECTS OF TEACHING

Rewards come to me in mentoring doctoral students to do research, and to publish their theory papers. Within the last few months, I moved on from another university, and I had a call this week from a student who I taught last fall and spring. She told me her theory paper was accepted for publication. I believe that there are 8 or 10 students who have published papers developed in theory classes. There was always other faculty members involved in supporting publication and I found this to be a very rewarding experience.

LEAST REWARDING ASPECTS OF TEACHING

I do not see things as least rewarding. Even circumstances that are really hard for me, and I am struggling; if I can stay with the struggle, eventually I can understand why I needed to do that. Usually the times that I stayed with the struggle are growth times for me. These times tell me a lot about myself and give me alternative ways to respond and to be in different situations. When things are difficult in any work situation, there is a tendency to separate from the difficulty, blame someone else, or ignore it. What I am suggesting is, that is it helpful to reflect on the situation enough to learn, but at the same time, not dwell on it to the extent that it hinders what you are doing. It is a balance. Least rewarding times cannot color the dimensions of who you are and how you are living. I have found that it is important to be with the struggle enough to decipher it. Be patient because you can never decipher difficult times all at once. Do it over time. I guess what I am describing is bigger than teaching. It is a way of living.

MAINTAINING EXCELLENCE AS A TEACHER

I have maintained excellence by keeping the links between theory, practice, and research. I really mean keeping them. I think that is where the uniqueness of nursing lives, in the intersection of theory, practice, and research. I believe I am most vibrant as a teacher when I am actually seeing patients, or when I am doing research and can apply my research in theory building. At these times, I am sharing with students in a way that makes sense to them. I think my excellence comes in being able to talk to a group of students in a research class and give them clear examples from what I am working on right now. That is what brings the didactic to life for me and for the students.

ADVICE FOR NEW TEACHERS

I suggest that teachers find out where the student is and stay where the student is. Try to stay there until you get in touch with them in a way that tells you how to move. I know that doing this is hard when you have a large class. It takes a bit of skill when you are working with a large class. Make sure you know where they are before you begin dosing them with ideas they are not prepared to understand. Do not underestimate the importance of getting a sense of where the students are. Another thing, be able to say that you do not know, but you will find out. Then, again, get very clear about where their question came from. I have found that students' questions reflect so much about who they are and where they are. I cannot always assume that I understand their question the first time I hear it. I ponder the question a little bit to make sure that I got it. I believe sometimes we act as if we understand the question, and move on too quickly. Try to fully understand where the students are by questioning the question. Try to understand what triggered the question. Do not take things personally. Recognize that when a student lashes-out and the lash out seems to be beyond the content of what has transpired, you are probably working with a student who has a complex history or a complex life situation. Try to stay on the course of what you are teaching. Do not disregard their anger, but perhaps address it later, rather than in the midst of a class. There will always be angry or disgruntled students no matter how good you are as a teacher. Teaching, for me, is a way of being present in every moment.

CHAPTER 11

E. Jane Martin

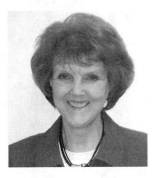

BACKGROUND

Dr. E. Jane Martin is Professor and Dean of the School of Nursing at West Virginia University. Dr. Martin earned a diploma in nursing from Mercy Hospital, a BSN Ed from West Virginia University, an MA in English from The Ohio State University, and an MN in Psychiatric Mental Health Nursing and a PhD in Higher Education from the University of Pittsburgh. She has postgraduate education in administration, mind-body medicine, and integrative cancer care. Dr. Martin is an experienced educator, having taught for over 30 years at the master's and doctoral levels. She is a Fellow in the American Academy of Nursing.

Dr. Martin is as an evaluator and trainer for the Commission on Collegiate Nursing Education (CCNE) and a deans' representative on the Accreditation Review Committee. She is also an elected member of the National Academies of Practice in Nursing and was a founding member of the American Holistic Nursing Association. Dr. Martin received the Distinguished Alumnus Award at the University of Pittsburgh. She served as editor of the *Journal of Holistic Nursing*.

STORY INTRODUCTION

Dr. E. J. Martin began her career in education by teaching English composition to undergraduate students. However, she chose to be an educator in nursing rather than in English and believes that being a teacher is a gift that has many rewards. Her career in teaching has been shaped by outstanding teachers, preparation in education and administration, and the challenge of finding balance in life.

EARLY INTEREST IN TEACHING

Although I was very aware in high school of what good teaching was and what it was not, it did not occur to me that teaching would be the path I would take. After high school I had a scholarship offer to go to a small college in Pennsylvania to become an art teacher. My art teacher had set it up without my input; it surprised me. I had no intention of doing such a thing, and when a person from the college talked to me about it, I said to him, almost indignantly, I am going to be a nurse. My high school teacher laughed afterwards and told me that I certainly set him straight. So, it had not occurred to me at that time that I wanted to be a teacher.

When I came to West Virginia University to do my bachelor's degree, the program for registered nurses was in the College of Arts and Sciences. Once in the program, I became very enamored while reconnecting with literature; I had loved it in high school. I took courses in arts and sciences and in English, so that I had an equivalent degree in English when I graduated with my nursing degree. Then I decided to pursue a master's in English at Ohio State University. There I received a Graduate Student Assistant (GSA) appointment and became a teacher overnight. An unprepared one, I must say. Every GSA was expected to teach freshman composition, a three-quarter sequence. There were thousands of students, so I taught three sections of freshman composition my first term in graduate school. I became a teacher the hard way.

We were all required to use the same books, follow the same syllabus, and make the same assignments. The structure was helpful, but no one told us how to teach in the classroom. So, I talked with people I knew who had some teaching experience, including my husband, who was a teacher. I got plenty of advice. My husband said, "Don't smile the first week," and then he said, "You can, perhaps, begin to smile a little bit the second week." We met three times a week with the students. It really was a trial by fire. I wanted to do a good job, and having three sections of the same course meant that I had three opportunities each week to work on it. I learned from each session, and I also learned that each group was different. Each group had its own personality. What worked in one group might not work in another in the same course. I also learned that first term what kind of trouble

I could get into if I didn't have clear guidelines and rules. In the first term, there was a lot of crisis intervention because I would be confronted with something and would not be sure how to handle it. I learned from that first experience. I went into the second quarter and had a much better sense about being very clear about ground rules, expectations, and consequences when expectations were not met. This helped a great deal to ease the turmoil of unhappy students. Each student wrote eight themes each quarter, and it was only a 10-week quarter. So they were writing from the get-go, and I had to grade each one. It was important that the papers came in on time so I could get them back to the students in a timely fashion. To complicate matters, I was taking six credits of graduate work, and I had two small children at home. It was an interesting life. I would talk with other people who were teaching and we would share stories about things that were happening.

I felt I really did acquire classroom teaching skills in the years teaching English at Ohio State. The first quarter focused on exposition—explanatory writing. The second was use of logic, judgment, and reasoning in writing. The third quarter was poetry, drama, and short stories. I loved the progression and learned about different types of writing, and how to help students work through the struggles of writing.

PREPARATION FOR TEACIIING

The first formal preparation was in my master's program; I took a three-credit curriculum course and also had a teaching practicum. In my doctoral program, I took a curriculum course and developed a curriculum in nursing; I took an evaluation course and developed an instrument to evaluate teaching. Every course I took, I brought back to nursing and made it fit. I would say most of my doctoral course work really did focus on education and enhanced my knowledge base and skills.

MENTORING FOR TEACHING

I have not had much formal mentoring. At Ohio State the director of the freshman program attempted to help. Probably the first person I could say really did mentor me was Dr. Marguerite Schaefer, who had been the Dean of Nursing at Pitt when I entered the master's program. After her deanship, she took a yearlong sabbatical and worked on organizational theory at Carnegie Mellon University (CMU) before joining the faculty in nursing administration. I took her courses in organization and management. She was absolutely an exquisite teacher who was incredibly respectful of students. She would always start her classes by clearing the agenda for any issue that was troubling people before she went on with the content of the course. I wanted to be a teacher like her. I could talk to her, not so much about teaching, but about my life and my career goals. She gave me very good feedback on written assignments. I would say she was the major mentor I had in teaching. She modeled what I wanted to be. Although she was friendly and available, she was not someone who was your buddy, but someone you could talk to about issues and concerns as a teacher.

After I completed my master's degree at Ohio State, I was hired as a lecturer while my husband was working on his PhD. At this time, our youngest daughter developed a stammering problem. I put her into speech therapy and the problem became worse, so I decided that what she needed was some time at home before she went to kindergarten, and I changed my teaching schedule. Ohio State had just received funding for a New Careers Program for adults in the community who needed academic course work, including writing skills, to prepare them for new employment opportunities. I was able to shift to that program, so that I could be home in the daytime with my daughter. Then my husband would come home from his commitments, and I would leave and do mine. It actually worked perfectly. My daughter's stammering problem cleared up, and when she began kindergarten, the teacher didn't even know she had ever had a problem. Teaching those adult learners was a challenge, and I greatly expanded my teaching skills. They had to be treated differently, and I needed different approaches to help them be successful.

I was careful to address these older students as Mr. or Mrs., and I helped them to understand that they knew more than they thought they knew. Most of them had had the benefit of a high school educational program that taught basic writing and grammar skills. In fact, these older students often had better basic skills than many of the freshman students that I taught. But, they needed confidence and were frightened about coming back to college. There was a tension between teaching them things they needed to know, and building on what they had already learned. I graded their papers differently, looked for different things in them, and tried to identify and emphasize their strengths. It seemed to work and was a very good experience for me.

We left Ohio State when my husband graduated, and we moved to Pittsburgh. I taught literature the first year in a small liberal arts college. Again, it was a different experience. I was teaching all levels of students, not just freshman or not just adult learners. While at this liberal arts college, I was a full-fledged faculty member. I marched in ceremonies, participated in events at the college, and I liked it all very much.

It occurred to me that I probably needed to get on with my education. I had a master's degree in English at that point, and I thought I had to either get a doctorate in English and continue in English, or, perhaps, return to nursing. My mother had always told me: "Being a nurse is like being a Catholic; once you are one, you are one the rest of your life, no matter what it is you are doing." To her, I was a nurse teaching English; I was not an English teacher who used to be a nurse.

I interviewed at the University of Pittsburgh in both the English Department and School of Nursing, and I decided that I would go back into nursing. I was fortunate to have funding, and I took classes on a full-time schedule in psychiatric mental health nursing. I completed a second master's degree and went straight into the doctoral program. That had been my intention when I went to Pitt. Following graduation with my master's, I was hired immediately on the faculty at Pitt. I taught the first term at the baccalaureate level, and then, because I had teaching experience, even though it was in English, they moved me to the master's level the second semester. So although I began teaching in a different field, the skills that I had acquired were useful and appropriate. The new learning was in clinical teaching. I had not done that before. However, as a student I had learned quickly what things were helpful from the faculty. Students figure out who the good faculty are, and who the not-so-good ones are. It seemed to me that the faculty who were good clinical teachers knew what they were doing because they also practiced. They were not hopelessly out of date. So, I had decided that as a teacher, I would need to practice, and when I interviewed for the position, I negotiated for time to practice as part of my workload. I saw patients at the nearby outpatient clinic and worked hours at the clinic around my teaching schedule. Practice gave me a rich repertoire of examples and illustrations, and I was walking the path I was asking students to walk. Then I began working with students doing research at the master's level. Learning how to guide students with their theses was also a new experience. Once I completed my own doctorate and became a member of the graduate faculty of the university, I moved on to doctoral teaching and worked closely with doctoral students through the whole curriculum. I found as I moved along in my teaching career that I began to do more presenting about teaching. My first publication was about teaching. It was application of a model in psychiatric nursing to teach psychiatric nursing students. Then a friend and I coauthored an article about incorporating standards of care into psychiatric mental health teaching.

I became distressed about the multiple degrees that were offered in doctoral education in nursing that seemed to me to be only adding confusion. I was "on the stump" for a number of years to have the only doctoral degree in nursing be the PhD. I wrote about it and presented at doctoral forums, but the PhD as the sole degree offered in nursing never happened.

FEELING COMFORTABLE AS A TEACHER

I think that by the third year of teaching at OSU, I was comfortable. By then I had learned that it was as much the student's responsibility to learn as it was my responsibility to teach, and I learned that in spite of planning and organizing, the perfect course could not occur. Flexibility was central to being successful.

CHALLENGES AS A TEACHER

The major challenge for me was the juggling of doing a good job in my teaching at the same time that I was either a student or faculty member and had a family to care for. I realized when I was at Ohio State, that unless I was willing to sacrifice my family life, I could not be a 4.0 student. I was studying for a master's degree in a field in which I was a "newcomer"; I did not have the rich background in English that some of my fellow students had. Many of the students were men, and school was their life's work. They had wives to take care of them, and they were very competitive. I had to make my peace with the fact that "Bs" were OK. I was not going to fail, but I just did not have to get an "A" in every course. As a GSA, I had to teach; I was learning to be a teacher, I had my children to care for, and my husband to support. So, it was a matter of doing some soul-searching and realizing that I did not have to be perfect in everything. It was a valuable lesson for me.

When I started my dissertation work, I enlisted my teenage children to help more at home. The girls would each take a turn cooking one night a week. Our agreement was that they would cook and we would eat, no matter what it was or how bad it was. They did—and we did. Incidentally, they are both wonderful cooks today. They also helped with some of the household chores. Asking for help was not always easy for me, but I learned to enlist other people's aid. Also, I learned to say "no" to things that I would have liked to do but just didn't have the time for. I still have trouble with saying "no" today; I want to do it all and be involved in as much as humanly possible.

Learning to prioritize was important for me at that time. I figured out that I was a morning person; I do my best work in the morning. So I got up every morning at 4:00 A.M. to work on my dissertation. I would always write in red ink. This was before computers, and to me the red ink was symbolic; it was blood. I was doing it; but it was not easy. I would write in the mornings until it was time to get the children up for school, and then after I came home from school and we had dinner, I would go back to the desk and would type what I had scribbled that morning. I knew that if I did not get it in a legible form, I would not know what I had written a week later. So, this became my routine for "grinding out the pieces" of the dissertation: getting up at 4:00 every morning and then trying to get to bed at a reasonable hour so I could get some sleep.

EMBARRASSING TEACHING MOMENTS

When I was teaching English, I had some dental work that required me to have braces on my teeth. The advice from my husband was to go in and smile the first day. It was not a usual thing in the early 1960s for adults to have braces, but I did it, and I let them see the full mouth of wires and rubber bands, and we went on from there. On one of the evaluations at the end of that term a student had written, "You are a very brave lady to appear in public like that." It was a compliment, I think. Another example, this one at Pitt when I was teaching in the master's program, is about a young student who had a baby and wanted to bring the baby to class. Of course I said she could. I learned later at the graduation celebration that the students were telling the story about one day when the baby began to fuss and the mother could not quiet the baby. So, at some point, I went back to the mother who was trying to give the baby a bottle. I shook the bottle, nothing came out, and I said, "Perhaps if there were a hole in the nipple, the baby could drink." I meant it kindly, and we got a pin and made a hole. At graduation, they were teasing me saying, "*Perhaps* if there were a hole in the nipple."

I do not know that I have ever been truly embarrassed in class. I think if you laugh at yourself, even if you do dumb things, it's not so embarrassing. It really makes you human, and that's OK.

REWARDING ASPECTS OF TEACHING

Probably one of the first rewards came when I was teaching at Ohio State. Many of the students were local farm kids and they did not have a very wide exposure to literature. So, for many of them, this was the first time they had a sense of what poetry, theater, and good fiction was about. I remember one woman, in particular, had turned in a very long evaluation that she had brought to class with her (rather than doing it in class as was customary). It was very moving, because she related that she had found in the work we had done that term new meaning and direction in her life. She was appreciative of the exposure and expected to continue to build on it. It was a very rewarding type of evaluation because that is really what most teachers hope for. You want to think that you are making a difference, that you are helping students see things in a new way, or a way that helps them come to some better understanding of their lives.

I learned that no statement is casual when you are a teacher. You never know what you say that a student will latch onto and that will sustain them. Another example relates to two women who came from India to the program at the University of Pittsburgh, and we faculty thought they would be just great buddies, since they were two women coming together from the same country. However, they were from different caste systems, so although they were together a lot, they were not good supports for one another because their cultures were very different. One of the women, in particular, had left a young child at home in India while she was in the program, and she suffered greatly because of it. When she was ready to graduate, she brought me a beautiful piece of cloth with gold in it. It was just gorgeous. I thanked her and said that she really did not need to do this. She said, "Oh, it is only because of you that I am finishing." And then she related that she had come to me once, asking if I thought she could to it; she was very unhappy and having great difficulty. She said, "You thought about it and then you said, 'I see no reason why you can't do this.'" She further explained that every time would say to herself, "I cannot do this," she would hear me say that there was no reason why she could not do it. I had told her that she could do it, and that was what sustained her. I am often amazed when I meet students later and they tell me that something I said to them had made such a difference. As educators, we never truly know the full effect that we have on people. Education makes a difference in people's lives. It is a wonderful thing that we do, and a wonderful thing that we are engaged in. To me those are the rewards.

LEAST REWARDING ASPECTS OF TEACHING

Least rewarding times are the failure to connect with or reach a student who needs some help or guidance. Once in a great while, you just cannot reach a student. My psychiatric nursing education has been valuable to me, and I am a better teacher because of that content. Once in a while, though, I find myself personally reacting to something, and that's a perilous path—most of the time a lose-lose situation. Although rare, for me, those are the times that are least rewarding, when I have just not been there for someone who needed guidance or help and it just did not go as well as it should have.

MAINTAINING EXCELLENCE

I subscribe to *The Chronicle of Higher Education* and read it to stay abreast of issues in education. I attend seminars and programs about new directions in teaching. I am particularly interested in where the field is going, perhaps where it ought to be going. I maintain excellence through reading more than anything else.

ADVICE FOR NEW TEACHERS

I would say that the opportunity to be an educator is a great gift that has the potential to make a profound and lasting contribution in the lives of people. It is important to approach the classroom with great courtesy and respect for every person present. I would say being a little more formal is probably better than being too informal and buddy-buddy with the students. They do not need friends. They have friends. They need a faculty member who is a role model who can take them to a place where they have not been before. I think it is important to have your course carefully thought out. To have your expectations clear and at the same time, be flexible. It is not easy to be flexible when you have it thought out and planned and you know where you are going. Knowing when to be flexible, and how you might then pick up the slack at another point in the course is a skill. It is important always to be fair and be consistent.

New teachers need to take time to write and talk about what they are doing and what they are learning as well as be open to new opportunities and experiences. I think one should take what sometimes might seem a different path, for a while, to see what might be found there.

I cannot say that there has been one book that has been like a "bible" for me that I would recommend to new teachers. I have recently purchased a copy of "Teacher" by Mark Edmondson. It is a story written by a student, whose life was changed profoundly by a teacher who came to his high school. It is a wonderful book. It vividly captures what an impact a teacher can have.

CHAPTER 12

Angela Barron McBride

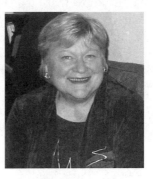

BACKGROUND

Dr. McBride received her bachelor's degree in nursing from Georgetown University, her master's degree in psychiatric-mental health nursing from Yale University, and her PhD in developmental psychology from Purdue University. She is a Distinguished Professor and University Dean Emerita at Indiana University School of Nursing. Dr. McBride has authored 4 books and has contributed to over 40 other books. She has published her work in over 70 professional journals and in several popular magazines.

Dr. McBride was given a Distinguished Alumna Award by Yale University and by Purdue University. She was elected as a Fellow of the American Academy of Nursing, and a Distinguished Practitioner of the National Academies of Practice, and was chosen to be a National Kellogg Fellow.

She received honorary doctorates from the University of Cincinnati, Eastern Kentucky University, Georgetown University, Medical College of Ohio, University of Akron, and Purdue University.

STORY INTRODUCTION

Dr. Angela Barron McBride has a deep commitment to facilitating career development of doctoral students and faculty in nursing. She believes that academic administrators maintain moral authority by continuing to teach and to publish. She views her relationship with Virginia Henderson as having a profound influence on her life.

EARLY INTEREST IN TEACHING

I don't know that I made a conscious decision to go into nursing education. When I finished my master's at Yale, I was invited to stay on and join the faculty. My decision to become a teacher was made for me in some ways because it was a very attractive environment. This was the decade of the 1960s, when the Yale School of Nursing was taking the lead in developing clinical research in nursing. Dickoff and James were at Yale writing about what it meant to be in a practice profession. It was an enormously stimulating environment. I shared an office with Donna Diers, next door was Jean Johnson and Rhetaugh Dumas, and Ernestine Wiedenbach and Elizabeth Sharp were on the other side.

The initial decision to take the teaching position was an opportunity that I thought I could not refuse. I worked full time at the beginning and found academia to be flexible when you had small children. Yale allowed me to work part time then, and I will always be grateful that I had interesting part-time work that was career building. So, I was not overwhelmed with juggling 3,000 things as a new mother. During my last years at Yale, I managed a National Institute of Mental Health (NIMH) grant focused on development of Psychiatric Nurse Institutes for Graduate Programs in the Northeast. There were 15 or 16 graduate programs involved in the grant. The Institutes were designed to take on cutting-edge topics in psychiatric nursing. It was a wonderful opportunity to think through new trends in psychiatric nursing. Much networking with leaders in that specialty was done during that time. I was fortunate to have a facilitative and understanding Department Chairperson, Rhetaugh Dumas, who was mindful of my career development (she was the Principal Investigator of the grant I managed). The faculty at Yale took their work very seriously and that really had a transforming effect on me. It helped me to take my work seriously and to become engaged with new developments in the field.

PREPARATION FOR TEACHING

There was no great push in that environment to get a doctorate; but there was a great push to do research and to publish. I subsequently got a doctorate at a Big Ten University and found that environment more concerned with making sure that you did all the right things on the way to the doctorate. In some ways the Yale environment had the notion that you were accomplished and expected you to go forth and do scholarship. It was an environment full of great expectations that has direct consequences for my thinking today. I am big on the importance of socialization. We sometimes do not challenge people enough, simply expect them to perform, and sort of run with it. Sometimes people surprise you in their capabilities if you stop fretting about what they can do.

When I was a master's student, there was the option, in addition to your clinical major, to also choose a functional area. It was possible to combine teaching and research so I took a clinical research course and a teaching course. The professor in the education course was an educational psychologist and I was probably his most difficult student. It was the least good grade I earned in my master's program because I found pedagogy extremely boring, and formulaic. I knew learning was not a formal process. It was engaging people in the possibilities of their field and in their work. I think I might have been too young for that course. I was still at the level of engaging students, while that course was aimed at the particulars of putting together a curriculum and lesson plans. I understood you needed some planning and ought to know what you were doing in class; but I found the course focused too much on pedagogy and not enough on the meaning of the subject matter. I must admit that I was a difficult pupil and did not show good will. What was driving my work was the development of clinical research and the excitement of the clinical field. So, I found a disconnect between the stilted nature of the pedagogy and the dynamic nature of what we were teaching. Clinical teaching made use of process recordings and reflective thinking about what was going on with patients; and that was the disconnect. Most of what the professor said pedagogically equated teaching with lecturing. Even his model for teaching about teaching was not relevant to how I thought I was going to teach.

MENTORING FOR TEACHING

I regard Virginia Henderson as my mentor, but she did not mentor me in ways currently considered mentoring. A mentor typically gives you tips, helps you with socialization, gives advice, recommends you for opportunities, and helps you move to the next level. That was not the way Virginia Henderson helped me. She helped me because she was open and interested in young people. I became a friend, saw what she did, and wrote chapter 49 for the last edition of *The Principles and Practices of Nursing*. We started working on that at least 8 years before it was in print. To see her thoroughness and her requirements for scholarship was enlightening. I remember giving her my chapter on the pain experience, which was a new chapter in the book. Previous editions had not focused on that topic, and my master's study had been on pain management. I remember getting the chapter done on time. And while she waited for other chapters to come in, she would regularly say to me, "Do you want to update it?" I thought I was finished and did not want to do anything more. She would keep after me to expand my work to include the latest literature and theories. I came to understand that she was a masterful individual, and she was the kind of thorough scholar I should aspire to be.

When I talk about mentoring, I think about it broadly. It is anything from a formal mentoring program to informal coaching/advising/counseling. I believe one has an obligation to facilitate the learning of subsequent generations. When a person is in a formal education program, he/she learns to read the lines. Mentoring and socialization experiences help one to read between the lines. The latter typically involves information that is not part of a formal education process. Students and new faculty need this type of mentoring. Schools of Nursing should be communities of learning, which means that everyone in that organization is learning and confronting what they do not know and need to get better at. A learning environment is one that is nurturing, and helpful in moving its members through key career transitions. My belief is that even curmudgeons have an obligation to mentor because that is part of what it means to be a professional in a community of learning. There is a whole literature on mentoring that is much more specific and talks about the components of formal mentoring programs. I believe it is equally important to encourage all to have a broad commitment to facilitate transitions and development of new generations.

EVOLUTION AS A TEACHER

My first position was as an instructor in psychiatric-mental health nursing, teaching graduate students. I was in my twenties and what I remember most vividly was the fact that I had a number of students who were older than I was. I was concerned about developing my own authority and style as a teacher, but I was relating to people who had considerably more life experience. Over time, I did adjust and got over being self-conscious, sort of the "imposter phenomenon" where you think your ignorance and ineptness is always on the verge of being exposed. I actually was the youngest member of the faculty for probably 2 or 3 years. Yale School of Nursing was then a youthful enterprise and many of us felt like pioneers; that sense of being in an exciting place went a long way in easing the awkwardness.

In the 1960s, you were unique if you had a master's degree and were expected to go forth and do good things. I handled many of my own anxieties and became part of that overall learning community by just talking to people who were more experienced than I was. I would stop by and chat with Virginia Henderson and others who were engrossed in their research. We would talk about a broad array of things. It was a time of listening to their thinking. The enrichment of our talks gave me confidence, and a sense of where I was headed, and where I wanted my students to be headed.

I would say that my next transformative period of change came after I earned a doctorate in developmental psychology, which complemented my background as a psychiatric nurse.

I obtained the PhD in 1978, and my first position afterwards was at Indiana University School of Nursing where I was hired to develop a doctoral program in psychiatric nursing. I arrived in the fall when the first doctoral students matriculated. They took core requirements the first semester, and the first course in the psychiatric nursing major was to begin in the second semester. I went on to develop all of the 15 credits in psychiatric-mental health nursing just one semester before teaching them. In the beginning, I also wound up being the main person delivering those 15 credit hours.

Designing a sequence of doctoral courses right after completing a doctorate was a challenge. The sequence was expected to prepare students to be able to do a really high quality dissertation in an area of concern to psychiatric-mental health nursing. At that point, I had done a great deal of broad reading about graduate education and the philosophy of science. I had already had experience with training grants, because I had written my own training grant for my doctoral program, which enabled me to get 2 years of support from NIMH. Indiana University had already obtained a training grant for the doctoral program in psychiatric-mental health nursing and I put the flesh on the bones, which I did with the help of a lot of experts. I have always been interested in effective people, figuring out how and why they are effective. I looked at what was good practice in education and psychiatric nursing, what prepared one to develop a program of research, then tried to do a replication.

DESIGNING THE FIFTEEN CREDITS
OF DOCTORAL STUDY

I had definite ideas about what should be included in the courses. There had been 14 years between when I earned my master's degree and doctoral degree. By this time, I had written several articles and two books and had grantsmanship experiences, so I had been productive and arrived full of ideas. The most important thing that I kept in mind in designing the courses was that I did not want any student to get to the point of dissertation unprepared. No one should ever get to her or his dissertation and say, "Now, what will I work on?" We would have failed completely if students were not prepared for the dissertation. So, that was the driving theme of the 15 credits.

The first 3-credit course focused on the history of psychiatric-mental health nursing, current trends, and broad concepts. If a person was being prepared to be a leader in psychiatric-mental health nursing, he/she should be knowledgeable about the past and have a sense of where the specialty is headed. The main assignment was that the students had to come to terms with what subject matter they were interested in studying for their dissertation. They had to do a critical review of the literature in that area, which could also serve as the literature review part of the dissertation. If everything went well in that course, students would be well on their way to completing the first chapter of the dissertation and would have developed the ability to do a critical review of the literature. Students read articles on what it meant to do a good critical review. The course sort of loosened up the student's thinking in understanding the practice problems that needed to be addressed.

In the second 3-credit course, students had to specify the phenomenon they were going to study, explore it in further for key concepts, and figure out the theoretical underpinnings that would guide their future work. For example, one student interested in family adaptation to childhood epilepsy immersed herself in models of family adaptation and attitude theory because she was interested in how attitudes shaped behaviors and adaptation.

In the third 3-credit course, students built on the work of the previous course and planned 6 credits of internship. The internship had two aims. Students were expected to implement and evaluate an intervention, and they were also expected to do some formal pilot work for the dissertation (e.g., testing the validity of an instrument never before used with this specific patient population). In order to do the pilot work, students had to go through all the clinical and research clearances, a process which was both time consuming and a great learning experience.

After completing these 15 credits, students then took 9–18 hours of dissertation credit. I am particularly proud of the fact that all of my dissertation students met my criteria for academic success, which is that they all presented their work at professional meetings and published their dissertation findings. At least half of the people whom I advised are now fellows in the American Academy of Nursing. I am very proud of their continuing success.

FEELING COMFORTABLE AS A TEACHER

Early on when I was doing clinical instruction with students at the Yale Psychiatric Institute, I changed the clinical experience from a model where the instructor sat waiting for students to have problems, to one where students managed patients and the instructor helped them use the resources of the setting in addressing problems. We relied on process recordings to help students think differently about ways of looking at what people were saying. The saving grace in both practice and research for me was that I have always been somewhat logical even before I had great skill. I was good at sorting out problems and thinking through approaches. When I was a fledgling teacher, there were no mentoring programs. Today, at least if a person came to my school, they would have mentoring as a junior faculty member and access to an array of both research and teaching opportunities.

CHALLENGES AS A TEACHER

Juggling work and family has been a challenge. I am married with children and grandchildren. For 12½ years, I commuted 125 miles round-trip. I have not lived and worked in the same community as my husband for 26 years. And, thankfully, I am married to someone who does not think this is a peculiar thing to do. When asked how I've managed, I cannot offer any answers. I managed these challenges differently in different decades. I made different decisions in different decades because it made sense. I could never have been University Dean of Indiana University School of Nursing with children still living at home with all the commuting and everything else. During the intense years of parenting, I held positions that allowed me to set some boundaries regarding my availability, which was not the case as dean. Juggling is difficult, but I have also turned that experience into an asset. I probably do more talks now about career development at different stages than anything else. In those talks, I remind the audience that there are no career opportunities in nursing that you have only once. Nursing is rich with opportunities. I encourage people to think through the fit between where they are in their personal lives and where they are career-wise. There is no one right way to handle living with contradictions; one of my books focused on the contradictions I've experienced as "a married feminist." I've actually used my own experience with "juggling" as a springboard for analyzing the growth and development struggles many women encounter, because these explorations fit with my professional identity as a psychiatric nurse.

EMBARRASSING TEACHING MOMENTS

I remember many awkward moments, but cannot think of a specific embarrassing situation in the classroom. I can give you my favorite story of being an after-dinner speaker. They wanted me to talk for an hour, which is not a wise thing to do after dinner. They seated me next to a man who was head of the Medical Center and who was near retirement. As soon as I started talking, he started sleeping. His snoring was not modest; it was loud and sawing. To add to the situation, as he snored, he shifted back and forth, and people were worried that he would fall off the chair. I talked for the requested hour; the applause at the end woke him up. He said goodbye on leaving adding, "You know that is the very best talk I've ever heard on women's health."

Another situation was an after-dinner speech honoring a retiring vice president for nursing. It was a good crowd and the wine flowed. As I talked, people did not stop talking among themselves. There were times when I would actually say, "Shhhhhh, they paid me to give this speech, and if you listen hard some of it is even funny." They would quiet down, then begin talking again. I kept shortening my remarks to get through the evening as quickly as possible. Thankfully, wine isn't served in the classroom, but evening classes can make for sleepy students!

REWARDING ASPECTS OF TEACHING

Being University Dean of the Indiana University School of Nursing provided me with wonderful opportunities to facilitate teaching, and that has been enormously rewarding, even more so than my personal success as a teacher. On the Indianapolis campus, we developed a Center for Teaching and Lifelong Learning, and we established new awards to honor master teachers and mentors statewide.

Every time a faculty member or graduate of the School gets into the American Academy of Nursing or receives some other honor, it is personal for me. That my colleagues are successful, particularly when they are honored for their teaching, I find enormously rewarding. My line used to be I want everybody in the building to be famous. One of the things I regularly asked in the annual review of the people who reported to me directly was, "What can I do to facilitate your career?" My goal was to make sure faculty had as much career success as possible because that would reflect on our school, and students would want to attend.

LEAST REWARDING ASPECTS OF TEACHING

When I think of my whole career, I think the last years of being University Dean were the "least rewarding." That was the case because the things that give me the most satisfaction were not as possible. During the years I served as University Dean, I necessarily became less engaged in my own field, because my time was taken in representing the School to the rest of the University and the larger community. My job was to keep the resources coming into the School of Nursing by helping the community understand that the School of Nursing was a treasure and having the University care about the School. I worked to make sure the President, Chancellor, and influential people with resources in the community understood that the School of Nursing was wonderful. So, I was heavily engaged in many activities that do not have immediate outcomes attached to them, or that do not provide the pleasure of associating with other nurses. You do a number of things that are "friend" raising in the hope that friend-raising will lead eventually to fund-raising.

MAINTAINING EXCELLENCE AS A TEACHER

Keeping up with your field is basic to maintaining excellence. One way to keep up is to teach. I taught a course every year that I was University Dean. This was very important because when you don't use skills you get scared to use them. One of my policies as University Dean was to say that no one was 100% in administration. I have seen people become administrators and do no teaching, then when they leave administration, they do not have a role in the school. They've lost the level of mastery necessary for teaching. I think it is very important, as an educational administrator, that one retains moral authority. Moral authority is kept when you continue to do, although not at the same level as other people, what other people are expected to do.

If an administrator is telling faculty to research, publish, and teach and they never see you do any of that, you really do lose credibility over time. People believe that you do not walk the talk. Keeping up with the growing knowledge base and doing presentations and publications are terribly important. Within 1 year of being at Indiana University, I became an administrator and was a Department Chair, then Associate Dean of research, and then University Dean of the school. So, how to keep up excellence along the way is something I've struggled with.

In the last 2 years of my career in administration, I got into so many things that keeping up became more difficult. For a time, I didn't publish anything professionally, which bothered me enormously. I did publish "think pieces" in our school's magazine, wrote grant proposals, and got increasingly involved in leadership positions in the community and in the university. I realized that if I worked all the time, it was getting impossible to do anything that was beyond what I had to do for the job. That was one reason why I decided to leave administration. After 23 years of academic administration, I decided that I wanted to do other things.

During the majority of those 23 years, I combined teaching and research in several ways. I developed a Women's Health course, which I taught for years. Then I wrote an institutional research training grant, for which I served as Program Director. We added a course to promote research socialization and anyone who was on the training grant had to take this course. I taught it annually for 13 years. The formal goals of the course were not unlike those of the first course in the psychiatric-mental health nursing program I had earlier developed, but the real goal was to inure the students to failure. By the end of the course, students knew that failure was to be expected and dealt with. To be successful in a career, the student had to learn to become like those sock-'em clowns that bounce back up when you punch them (the "punch" typically is being told that your work is not yet the incarnation of perfection). All students were expected to put together a 3-year statement regarding their research goals. Students regularly said that to get the degree was their goal. My response always was that if the only thing we did was to give students a doctorate, we failed. We wanted additional outcomes along the way. Students also wrote a contract in which they customized their objectives. If students were at the beginning of a program, they might decide to do a critical review of literature. Or, this might be the course where they wrote a grant proposal to obtain funding for their dissertation research. One of the things students often did was to think through whether there was something they had done in their doctoral studies that could be turned into a publishable paper. I urged the class to aim for outcomes and not just a degree, for example, refereed presentations/publications. We even role-played job interviews, particularly the art of self-presentation.

These days, a leader should have favorite websites. If you have a research idea and you are going forward to get funding, you should know the strategic plan of the funding agency you plan to approach. If the National Institute on Aging has priorities, then you as a geriatric nurse ought to know about those areas. Guest lecturers in my course were consequently asked to talk about their favorite websites. Related to that, I have found it to be effective in teaching people to handle failure to have guest lecturers discuss the failures they've experienced. Students typically look at the successful and assume they've always been successful. The successful, however, are people who got a score on a grant application, knew that they had to redo most of the application as a result of the feedback and they maybe even received a worse score the next time, and then redid that one too. If you think anyone who is successful was just successful without hassles, chances are you simply do not know them well enough. What doctoral students need to understand is how really successful people developed a program of study, how they went about focusing on an area, and how they then worked to become successful over time.

ADVICE FOR NEW TEACHERS

There are two pieces of advice I would give. One is to really confront the notion of who is the "real nurse." We still have residual stereotypes that shape the whole field. For example, if you are not at the bedside, you are assumed not to be a real nurse. Therefore, someone who is an educator may not be considered to be a real nurse. New teachers should take this stereotype and turn it around. What this requires is to see the connection between what you are doing, that is, teaching, and real nursing. I used to take great umbrage when somebody would say to me as dean, "Tell me about when you used to be a real nurse." I would fluff up my feathers and go on, at great length, to tell them about the connection between what I was doing right now and what real nursing was about. There was a direct relationship between what I was doing and whether there would be a workforce of prepared nurses in the United States. We are more and more becoming knowledge workers. New teachers should understand that they are an important part of mainstream nursing.

The second thing is that you never know what influence you have on students. In a spirited discussion in class, you can have fun, end the course, and have enjoyed it. In teaching there is a lot of immediate satisfaction, but there are some satisfactions that you are not prepared for and they are even more wonderful. What touched me most was when I was at a professional meeting and a former student told me how I had influenced her life. This individual had been chatty in class, but did not know how to develop her ideas in depth. In her final evaluation, I told her she was a fuzzy thinker. It turned out that she was on drugs, and, at the time, thought it did not show. The fact that I told her she was a fuzzy thinker made her realize that it did show, and that was the beginning of her recovery. I have forevermore been empowered to tell people they are fuzzy thinkers when that is the case. I believe most nurses who are educators have a few stories like that.

CHAPTER 13

Diana Lynn Morris

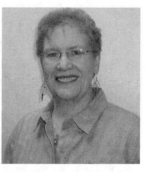

BACKGROUND

Dr. Diana Lynn Morris is an Associate Professor of Nursing and Associate Director for Programming at the University Center on Aging & Health, Case Western Reserve University. She earned an Associate Degree in nursing from Point Park College, a bachelor's degree in nursing from Pennsylvania State University, and a master's and PhD in nursing from Case Western Reserve University. She is a Fellow in the American Academy of Nursing and is a past recipient of a National Institute of Mental Health (NIMH) Faculty Scholar Award in Geriatric Mental Health with a focus on long-term care residents.

Dr. Morris has received an Award of Appreciation from the master's in nursing science students at the University of Zimbabwe; the National League for Nursing Lucile Petry Leone Award for Teaching Excellence; and the Elizabeth Russell Belford Founders Award for Excellence in Education from Sigma Theta Tau International. Dr. Morris's research interests include self-care in elderly family caregivers, geriatric mental health, the health of minority elders, and training of formal and informal caregivers. She has authored numerous book chapters and is published widely in refereed nursing journals.

STORY INTRODUCTION

Dr. Morris's story is a journey in learning and teaching, from the bedside to the university classroom, from rural America to Africa. She believes that a large part of her success derives from her early teachers and strong mentors throughout her practice and teaching career.

EARLY INTEREST IN TEACHING

My first teaching experience was in first grade when Mrs. Varnham, my first grade teacher, asked me to help others with their reading. I was able to read before going to school because my grandmother had taught me to read and do math before I went to first grade. Even though my grandmother had to quit school and go to work, she valued education and encouraged us to learn. We had a special shelf in the living room for our books. She would encourage us to role-play; I would pretend to be a newspaper reporter, store clerk, preacher, or teacher. We always talked about things going on in the community and news with my grandparents and parents. We were not excluded like some young women were. My grandparents had all girls and then my parents had girls, and we were always part of the discussion.

Teaching others to read in first grade was a special experience for me. It made me feel good to be able to help. My desire to learn and help others learn also was reinforced by my participation in Bible School and the teachers there.

Another important experience occurred in high school. I had a teacher who believed in mastery, so when I finished one book she had others to recommend. You could move on even if the other students were not ready to do so.

My early interest in teaching nursing occurred when I was a student in an Associate Degree nursing program. I thought that quality nursing care was not being provided to the patients. At that point I thought I would like to teach because, as a nurse educator, I could make a difference in nursing care.

My interest in teaching nursing was reinforced when I was a nurse manager, working with staff and trying to support their development. I was a nurse manager at 21 years old, when I was too young to know that I should not be. I began taking management and general education courses so that I could do a better job with staff development. While in this leadership role as a nurse manager, I had an idea of the content that I wanted to present but I did not know much about how to deliver the content. I did not know about curriculum development or educational design. So I signed up for workshops and some formal classes as well. I also worked closely with an experienced teacher from the nursing education office who could provide guidance and supervision for my teaching. As a manager, I was further influenced to think about teaching by a nursing professor from a local university who had students on my unit and also by one of the staff development faculty. Both of these individuals kept telling me that I was a very good manager but that they thought my calling was teaching.

My first formal teaching experience was soon after I finished my baccalaureate degree. I had a clinical teaching position, supervising the clinical learning of RN to BSN students. I then took a teaching job at a diploma school, and was using that to pay for my master's degree education. So, I was using the content I gained in workshops to prepare myself in topics such as curriculum development, testing students, designing courses, designing objectives properly, and lesson planning. I also was working with colleagues who were known as excellent classroom and clinical teachers, so that I observed and interacted with quality role models. I selected those who had expertise in the areas that I needed to develop, such as clinical teaching and test construction.

PREPARATION FOR TEACHING

When I enrolled for the baccalaureate degree program at Penn State I was in one of the early external degree programs in the western part of the state. I enrolled for general education courses as part of my elective credits in the BSN program. I also continued to participate in education workshops and continuing education focused on teaching. When I was in Pittsburgh I participated in a number of workshops focused on the dynamics and artistry of engaging learners, and the process of interaction in the classroom. These workshops were not just about how to create a course outline or structure an exam, but rather they were focused on the mutual interaction between faculty and student, and the teacher's use of self as a tool in the classroom.

I was teaching full time and was studying for my master's degree part time. I continued to participate in workshops designed for nurse educators that were offered in the local community. One of the workshop faculty members was Dr. Litwak, who had been at Kent State. He was conducting many workshops around curriculum development. In addition, my master's degree program included a focus on educational principles, as it was a psychiatric nursing curriculum designed to prepare clinical specialists. The courses included change theory and adult learning principles. Components of educator preparation focused on adult learning, change theory, staff development, and management were all part of the preparation for clinical specialists for indirect services to support quality care.

One of the books that I read at that time, recommended by the director of the psychiatric nursing program, was *Teaching as a Subversive Activity*; it is one of the most outstanding books I have ever read on teaching. It includes a focus on the Socratic method and emphasis on the fact that the teachers' questions are not as important as the students' questions. Another book that influenced me was one by Litwack and Wykle, focused on counseling and clinical supervision of students. It is the best thing I have ever read in this area of educator preparation. I still recommend it to graduate students. I was already interested in teaching and had been doing teaching, but this graduate education provided an opportunity for me to integrate the learning.

MENTORING FOR TEACHING

I have absolutely been mentored in teaching. I did not know it then, but I was mentored by one of my first faculty members, Helen Wright, who taught me in the Associate Degree nursing program. I had grown up in a rural community and did not know much about the world; she told me I could be a leader. She took me under her wing and started to expose me to the larger community, and to various roles and ways I might participate in the community. She was a role model and a mentor to me.

My main mentor has been May Wykle. In fact, I came to Case because I had met May at some staff development classes she was presenting. I decided I wanted to study with her and learn to be a therapist from her. I also learned about teaching from her because I worked for her as a graduate assistant. This position included formal teaching as well as participation on research and training proposals and grants. I learned about curriculum development and innovative programming while preparing training proposals with May, working with the grant supported students, and developing clinical sites to support the curriculum.

EVOLUTION AS A TEACHER

My teaching has evolved so that I now approach the process in terms of working with and thinking about the interaction with students. I not only consider this interaction in clinical teaching but also in working with them in the classroom. My teaching style is informed by what I learned as a psychiatric nurse and by the clinical supervision that I had in my own educational program. I have used that kind of clinical supervisory process as a teacher, where I seek out a master teacher to be a supervisor to me. I use this process as I would if I were in a therapy role, to monitor myself in terms of how I am relating to students, and to determine if I have too much energy around some issue and may have my own theme interference or bias. Talking to someone in a supervisory capacity is part of my own learning and development. I have also continued to enroll in workshops and continuing education courses to assist me in thinking about different ways of designing courses and different approaches to teaching. Even at research conferences if there are papers presented on education that I think will be helpful, I will attend these presentations.

FEELING COMFORTABLE AS A TEACHER

I was comfortable teaching in a clinical setting and supervising students in clinical experiences within a couple years after I started teaching. Initially, I had a much greater comfort level with clinical teaching because I felt very comfortable with my knowledge in my specialty area. Also, having been a manager in the clinical setting helped me to feel comfortable in clinical teaching. In the classroom, I am not sure exactly when I began to feel comfortable, but it was some time during my master's degree program when I was teaching part time. Probably it was 3 to 4 years after I started teaching that I became comfortable in the classroom. I think I was mature enough that it was alright with me if I did not always have the answers, or if students raised issues that I had not already addressed. Even now when I am preparing a new course, and presenting it for the first time, there is some discomfort; but not like it was when I first started teaching. The discomfort comes from knowing that if it is something new, it may not exactly work the first time, and that is OK. You work through it and you work with the students, and you resolve any questions that might occur. You identify what is working and what is not working. As a teacher, one reaches a maturity level where any difficulties or problems are not perceived to be personal inadequacies but part of the process of evaluation and course development. It is important to invite the students to join in the process. I try to do that every time I start a class. I communicate to the students that this is their class, and I am there as a resource. When I was younger in teaching, or just younger in terms of my career in general, even though I did some inviting of student input, I was not as comfortable with it.

CHALLENGES AS A TEACHER

Some of my most significant challenges have been related to facilitating students' growth. A couple of students I have had in classes decided they were just marking time and they either already knew the content or they did not need to know it. In fact, there is always the potential to grow. I have to be careful because I think sometimes (more often in the past), if I am not careful I start to get frustrated and sometimes angry in situations where my perception is that a student does not wish to learn. That is a difficult situation. I think I manage it better than I used to because I try to focus on what I can do to make the situation different. Yet, maybe sometimes there is nothing I can do. I need to let that person just be where he or she is, even if it is not where I would like the person to be.

EMBARRASSING TEACHING MOMENTS

I went to do a class on interpersonal relations and professional relationships that I was teaching for nutrition graduate students. I had been hurrying in my morning preparations. I did not have my glasses on when I got dressed and when I got into the classroom I had on two different shoes. There are other times when I am talking about something and the wrong word comes out. For example, one time I was trying to say circumscribe and I said circumcised. It was with a younger group of students, so they thought that was pretty funny, and that I was pretty much an idiot. I am the one that always edits things, and I have my technical equipment, but I do not always follow the detailed steps well enough not to make or correct editing mistakes. So when I do err, I have to beg for patience from some students who want it perfect. They equate mistakes with the faculty member not being organized or prepared.

REWARDING ASPECTS OF TEACHING

I enjoy teaching more each year. It is more fun partly because it is less stressful. I have had more experiences with a variety of students in a variety of settings, dealing with different information and different resources. Besides the structured evaluations the students do for the University, I always ask them, no matter what level student they are, to do a narrative self-evaluation. It is rewarding to see different things that emerge from the learning that occurs in students. When they really get something about what you were hoping to communicate, or they really understand, it is rewarding. For example, in the aging course that I teach one of the greatest things is having new students gain insight into the relationship between culture and health or the humanity of those they care for. They would say things like, "One of the things that I learned is, I really have to listen to people and pay attention. I am not just taking care of the equipment." It is not so much a singular event, but the change in students caused by events. If you can facilitate that learning, it is rewarding.

LEAST REWARDING ASPECTS OF TEACHING

Some of my least rewarding times were when I got frustrated when other teachers labeled students who asked questions as deviants. That was frustrating to me, and it is still frustrating even though I think I am more mature now and do not always interpret this in an antagonistic way. I try to understand the perspective of the other teachers, yet sometimes I still have to be righteously indignant. From my perception this type of response to students does not allow them to reach their potential. It closes off the options for students' learning, and that is frustrating for me. I particularly saw this happen at the diploma school where I taught; students who asked questions were perceived negatively. They were not deviant; they often just had more creative ideas and a great curiosity. The attitude of the other teachers made it easy for me to decide to leave there, even though I was not sure what my next position would be and there was a benefit that was helping to pay for my graduate education.

MAINTAINING EXCELLENCE AS A TEACHER

I think the most important thing that one can do is to grow as an educator. This can be accomplished by going to workshops and seminars. Also, I learn from each class I teach. I always use some more experienced faculty member as a colleague-supervisor who can help me process how I am doing. I think that it is important for the educator to be a lifelong learner. Also, the professional behaviors that we encourage among our students are relevant for us as faculty as well; i.e., it is important to continue to develop self-awareness and understanding. Invite others to give you feedback and listen to the feedback that you are given. For me part of the development of excellence is to continue to play with ideas and focus on interactions with students as they learn—the "ah-has." The mutual interaction between students and faculty is important to me; it challenges me to keep thinking and to keep looking for something new. I am always learning something from the students on hearing another perspective I have not heard before; that keeps me energized.

ADVICE FOR NEW TEACHERS

One of the most important things new teachers can do is to recognize that teaching is not a one-way street. The teacher must be a lifelong learner, not only in your particular area of expertise, but also in how you think about teaching. Know also that you will make mistakes. You will edit things incorrectly. You do not have to have all the answers. It is actually good to let students know you do not have all of the answers, but that you can teach them how to seek answers and solve problems for themselves.

CHAPTER 14

Adeline Nyamathi

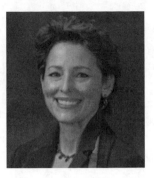

BACKGROUND

Adeline Nyamathi is Professor and Associate Dean for Academic Affairs at the University of California, Los Angeles School of Nursing. She earned the BSN at Hunter College Bellevue School of Nursing, MSN at State University of New York at Stony Brook, and PhD from Case Western Reserve University. She is a Fellow in the American Academy of Nursing and has received numerous teaching awards over the course of her career.

Dr. Nyamathi is responsible for organizing and implementing educational programs locally and internationally. Her funded research has been directed at assessing the effectiveness of health education and resource programs among homeless and impoverished populations. She is presently conducting an investigation in one of the largest Indian System of Medicine programs in Delhi, where there is an integration of HIV education and prevention. She is widely published on works related to HIV/AIDS.

STORY INTRODUCTION

Dr. Nyamathi believes that teaching, research, and administration is a wonderful and very fulfilling academic role combination. Along with her administrative responsibilities, she teaches courses in the doctoral program on the state of the science in family and community research, and maintains a continuous engagement in funded research projects. Although she did not participate in a formal mentoring program, she learned much from her teachers. She guides new faculty to seek the resources that they will need to help them become the best that they can be.

EARLY INTEREST IN TEACHING

I first became interested in teaching after I had completed my master's program and was in the doctoral program. The idea of working in an academic setting and doing research was very appealing to me.

PREPARATION FOR TEACHING

I went through the Francis Payne Bolton School of Nursing Program at Case Western Reserve University. We did not have any formal classes on how to teach and this is why it was very important for me to offer education courses to our doctoral students. We offer a special course where students are enrolled in a four-unit course and spend 10–12 hours a week with a faculty member who is engaged in teaching. They help the faculty member develop the course objectives and the exams for the class, including evaluating the psychometric properties of the exams. The students also provide lectures in the class as well as sit in and observe the expertise of the faculty member.

MENTORING FOR TEACHING

We did not have mentors in the doctoral program I attended; however, at the UCLA School of Nursing, I learned from the people who inspired me. These are teachers who have impressed me greatly in terms of their ability to engage students, while being humble. They were able to provide a wealth of information and inspire students to become wonderful in their own right, and to achieve the goals they had envisioned for themselves. It is these people whom you emulate and strive to model in your teaching.

EVOLUTION AS A TEACHER

My expertise has evolved over time in that I am becoming less rigid. I have always been good at listening to students and learning from them. Over time, you become more expert in your area of research and the theoretical constructs that you teach. It almost becomes second nature, so that you could do it in your sleep. When one becomes so engaged in research, then the actual practice of what you do makes the teaching much more natural and full of examples and illustrations that really provide depth and quality to the experience of teaching.

My research is situated in Los Angeles and in India. In Los Angeles, I have been an NIH funded researcher for 17 years; and have focused on improving the health and well-being of homeless populations. What we have done in 17 years is to provide intervention programs, where we enroll homeless adults in an intervention or a usual care program. We educate them about HIV risk reduction and health promotion activities, and evaluate the impact of the intervention when it is 6 months, 1 year, or 2 years out. We have engaged a wonderful group of nurses who are very much a part of the community where we work. The community is called Skid Row. It is where the homeless pitch their tents and cardboard box condos. It is where they live on the streets and where they function. Our staff is situated there and I go out and have meetings with them taking part in the research side by side with them as often as I can. The clients/participants involved in our program have known the staff for many years and are always interested in knowing what will be our next grant. They help us in terms of being a reality check as far as where we are going next. We have expanded our HIV prevention focus to include TB and hepatitis prevention. Currently, we enroll homeless adults who are TB positive into a TB prevention program. These people have all been exposed to TB, are not active yet, but are much more likely to become active TB patients because they have poor immune systems, improper diets, are into drugs and alcohol, and live in very close quarters. All the factors place them at high risk for acquiring active TB. In this study homeless adults are enrolled in a special nurse case managed program or usual care, and are paid a nominal amount of money to receive twice weekly INH medication for 52 weeks. We had 72% in this special nurse case managed program complete TB chemo-prophylaxis, compared to 46% in the control group. They both were paid the same amount of money, so it was not the money. It was engaging with nurses who really cared for them and encouraged them to come to the program.

The courses I teach in the doctoral program relate to the state of the science in terms of family and community research. They very much focus on what I do in my day-to-day activity with research. We talk about ways to engage the community and becoming culturally competent. I teach three doctoral classes and am the Associate Dean, thus part of my time is spent in administration.

Teaching, research, and administration are a wonderful combination. I interact with the faculty in revising the curriculum, keeping the curriculum up to date, and minimizing redundancies throughout the program. I bring culturally competent experiences to the faculty and to the program. For example, just today I interviewed someone who is interested in offering a Spanish immersion class in Mexico. I am part of the Dean's advisory committee, so we discuss budget and many related issues.

FEELING COMFORTABLE AS A TEACHER

I've been teaching since 1984, and would say after about 5 or 6 years that I fell into a niche about what I really love to talk about and teach.

CHALLENGES AS A TEACHER

The challenges that I face relate to being competent in fulfilling the many activities faculty have to do at the same time. Not only are they expected to be expert teachers, but also to be prosperous with a program of research. Faculty have to write grants, and write manuscripts. The challenge becomes how to juggle all these activities at the same time while grading papers and being available for students any time of the night or day.

EMBARRASSING TEACHING MOMENTS

One time I was teaching about the cardiovascular system and was talking about ejection fraction and used the term ejaculation by mistake. My husband who is a cardiac surgeon always reminds me of that one.

REWARDING ASPECTS OF TEACHING

The most rewarding outcomes of teaching are seeing students grow. To engage them when they are so unsure of themselves and lacking in self-esteem, then to watch them progress, and see how well they do with a little bit of advice and recommendation is marvelous. Watching how students just take off is the most rewarding experience for the faculty. We have also been able to get the students involved in our research and use this involvement as a teaching opportunity.

LEAST REWARDING ASPECTS OF TEACHING

I have not experienced any unrewarding aspects. However, I am sure that there are faculty who do experience times that are not rewarding. One situation that I know of is about a very brave faculty member who is really pushing hard to get the students to have excellent writing skills. The students come in with diverse writing skills and for her to push the students to rewrite their papers is a challenge. Students can become hostile about these kinds of things. It is frustrating for me to hear how the students really blasted her in her evaluation. However, several students reported that the course had made them become better writers.

MAINTAINING EXCELLENCE AS A TEACHER

I maintain excellence by continuing to do all the activities that I do. By this I mean continuing to engage in research, getting the experiential background to constantly be involved in teaching, and always striving to be an excellent teacher. I am still growing and continuing to learn from people that I admire as teachers.

ADVICE FOR NEW TEACHERS

First of all, faculty have to be aware of all the available resources in the school and on the campus. For example, there is instructional support for faculty where they can learn how to do PowerPoint and how to deal with large classes, hostile students, and disruptive students. We have a mentored approach with young faculty when they first join the faculty. They are paired with a more senior and experienced faculty member. The new faculty member can sit in on classes of the more experienced faculty member, ask questions, and be guided in terms of teaching. More importantly, they are guided in terms of moving along the tenure process, because that is where the faculty oftentimes get hung up or do not progress very well. This mentorship really functions on all levels in teaching and also research. We also have an Associate Dean for Research who helps faculty in terms of reviewing their grants and making sure their grants are ready to be submitted to NIH. We have modeling parties where faculty function similarly to an NIH review study session, giving sound advice to the faculty member before the grant goes out. Because I am an endowed chair, along with two other faculty, we are going to be offering these Faculty Research Oriented Groups (FROG), where we engage the faculty who are writing manuscripts. There are all different kinds of resources that faculty need to seek. Thus my advice is to go out and seek the resources that they need to help them become the best they can be.

CHAPTER 15

Marilyn Oermann

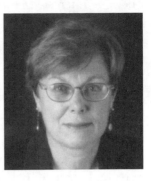

BACKGROUND

Dr. Marilyn Oermann received her undergraduate degree in nursing from Pennsylvania State University, a master's degree in nursing from the University of Pittsburgh, and a PhD from the University of Pittsburgh in curriculum and instruction. Dr. Marilyn Oermann is a Professor in the College of Nursing, Wayne State University, Detroit, Michigan.

She is author/coauthor of 10 nursing education books and more than 150 articles in nursing and health care journals. Her current books are *Writing for Publication in Nursing, Evaluation and Testing in Nursing Education,* and *Clinical Teaching Strategies in Nursing Education. Evaluation and Testing in Nursing Education* received an American Journal of Nursing Book of the Year Award and a Best Books of the Year Award.

Dr. Oermann has written extensively on educational outcomes, teaching and evaluation in nursing education, and using the Internet to teach consumers about quality care. She is the Editor of the *Annual Review of Nursing Education* and *Journal of Nursing Care Quality,* and a Fellow of the American Academy of Nursing.

STORY INTRODUCTION

Dr. Oermann is well known and regarded for her presentations and writings on curriculum, instruction, and evaluation in nursing education. Her story is one of a career dedicated to scholarship in nursing education. She has influenced many students of nursing education over the years, through her formal courses and continuing education programs, as well as through her many publications in the area of nursing education.

EARLY INTEREST IN TEACHING

I became interested in teaching when I was doing clinical teaching at the University of Pittsburgh. That was my first position and was back in the days when you could get a master's in nursing education. When I was a practicing nurse, I did a lot of patient teaching and worked with students on the unit. Teaching seemed like something I would be good at.

PREPARATION FOR TEACHING

I earned a master's in nursing education and a minor in medical-surgical nursing. I had a lot of courses in nursing education and back then, people were very well prepared in these programs. They were long master's programs; instead of the clinical specialty focus, the focus was nursing education. I went on and earned a doctorate in curriculum and evaluation. At that time there were very few nursing programs at the doctoral level. While at the University of Pittsburgh in my doctoral program, the University had just been funded for a center for research on learning and instruction. So instead of this being a typical education program that focused on pedagogy, it focused on research. The program had a strong thread of scholarship. Your role as an educator was as a scholar doing research.

Between my master's and my doctorate I taught 1 year, replacing Sister Rosemary Donley, who left Pitt and went to Catholic University. That was a good experience. I taught at the baccalaureate level and also one master's level course. I found that I was actually very good at lecturing. Back then we did all lecturing. I was well organized and liked lecturing. I had a good style of teaching and wanted to teach. However, I did not want to teach in a diploma or technical program.

After my doctorate, I went to Wayne State. Dorothy Reilly was there. She was kind of the guru of nursing education. She had written a lot of books. I had very good mentoring.

MENTORING FOR TEACHING

I was mentored early in my teaching career by people who were experts in teaching at the University of Pittsburgh. They had a nursing education program and a cadre of faculty, many of whom were prepared as teachers. Sr. Rosemary was one of my first mentors. She and Sr. Mary Albert Kramer coordinated the nursing education program and were prepared in evaluation and testing. When I moved to Wayne State, I worked with Dorothy Reilly who had done a lot of writing and ran a continuing education department. She also taught the nursing education courses. Again, that program was a master's level nursing education program. All three of these nursing educators were my mentors.

EVOLUTION AS A TEACHER

My evolution as a teacher has come from experience and from doing a lot of writing. When you do a lot of writing and a lot of reading, you ask questions about what other people are doing. My teaching evolved when I had a new course to teach and worked on the research needed to carry it through. I would go to the research in another field and say, "Now here is new research; how can we use that in nursing?" This is the basis for a lot of books and articles I write now.

FEELING COMFORTABLE AS A TEACHER

I felt comfortable after about 2 years into my doctoral program. I had already had my master's in nursing education and had some experience as an educator. In addition I worked with a mentor where the preparation was put in place.

CHALLENGES AS A TEACHER

Teaching inadequately prepared students is a challenge. That goes across all settings and all courses. I see it today, not in terms of nursing education, but in lack of preparation to do the thinking that is needed to be a scholar and in the lack of preparation in writing. In my early career, there was the challenge of balancing clinical teaching, classroom teaching, service, publishing, and research in the academic role. I think people still have that problem today.

EMBARRASSING TEACHING MOMENTS

In one of my courses Madeleine Leininger was a guest lecturer and her responsibility was to talk about cultural aspects of teaching. She brought the wrong notes. What she covered had nothing to do with teaching, and the students kept looking at me. Nevertheless, Madeleine did a great job sharing her expertise. About 2 years after that, I was giving a guest lecture and had the wrong notes and the wrong slides. I just turned off the projector and did it by heart.

REWARDING ASPECTS OF TEACHING

The last 10–15 years have been most rewarding. In the 1980s universities started to close nursing education programs. At Wayne State, when they voted to close the program, the Dean told me, "If you want to prepare for nursing education, then do something." Instead of saying, "We voted and you're out," she in turn said, "Whatever you want to do, go ahead." The University at that time had started giving a post-master's certificate. I went to the Provost and discussed a post-master's certificate in nursing education. She told me to write a proposal, which was approved. The program started in 1989. By 1995, the market was saturated and basically everyone in metropolitan Detroit had taken these courses. I then decided to shift to Web-based courses. No one had ever done a Web-based course at Wayne State. The Dean gave me release time and hired an instructional designer. I did each course gradually semester by semester. Now since 1997, you can take the nursing education courses once a month on a Saturday face to face, or as a Web-based course completely on-line. Last year, I found that students do not really want to take the course on-line if they live in the local area. They want to be present with the teacher, sit for coffee, and talk about educational issues. Last year I started offering both versions at one time. I tell the students, if you want face-to-face and cannot come one of the Saturdays, you can go to the on-line version. This has been a really good idea. I have full enrollment and a waiting list in every course. I have a Navy nurse in Japan, a student from Vancouver, and a student from Arizona. I could probably get more international students, but it takes time to do the marketing, and I do not have the time. I think this has been a rewarding period.

LEAST REWARDING ASPECTS OF TEACHING

In the 1980s when I was working part time and trying to develop a career as a part time faculty, I found it was nearly impossible. I found that people are not very supportive of faculty who are not full time.

MAINTAINING EXCELLENCE AS A TEACHER

I have maintained my excellence through writing, speaking, and finding new ideas in other fields. I have tried out new approaches like the Web-based and the post-master's programs. These activities have contributed to my excellence as a teacher.

ADVICE FOR NEW TEACHERS

New teachers need to be prepared educationally for their role. They should not take a job unless they will be provided with faculty development. We set teachers up for failure by hiring them for courses when they have no experience in teaching. For example, they have to give a lecture and they have never given a lecture. New teachers should learn to say no. New teachers should allow time in their role for scholarship because otherwise it will be the kiss of death when it comes time for getting tenure. I would encourage new faculty to get involved in faculty development, to take a course, or a workshop. Eventually, I would like to take the post-master's courses and package them into modules for faculty development. In the course I teach on clinical teaching there is one class on assessing a clinical agency before you take students, one module on how to work with staff, and a couple of classes on clinical evaluations. These could be offered on-line for faculty development. On-line courses are the wave of the future for faculty development. They can be taken in one's own time because they are self-paced.

New faculty should find a good mentor. Your teaching mentor may not be the same as your research mentor. New faculty must search out a mentor; the mentor is not going to come to them.

CHAPTER 16

Lynn Rew

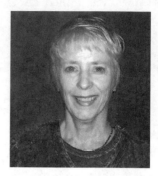

BACKGROUND

Dr. Lynn Rew received her baccalaureate degree in nursing from the University of Hawaii, a master's degree in community health nursing from Northern Illinois University, and an EdD from Northern Illinois University in counselor education. She completed a postdoctoral fellowship at the University of Minnesota in adolescent health. She is Professor, School of Nursing, University of Texas at Austin, and Director of the Southwest Partnership Center for Nursing Research on Health Disparities.

Dr. Rew's scholarship focuses on sexual health in adolescents. She is currently funded to do a 3-year study of sexual health practices of homeless adolescents. She is certified both in psychiatric and holistic nursing, and serves as the editor of the *Journal of Holistic Nursing*. Dr. Rew is widely published in the nursing literature, primarily in the areas of adolescent health and health risks among vulnerable groups.

Throughout her career as a nurse educator, Dr. Rew has encouraged a number of nurses to pursue careers in research, through her mentoring and advisement and her role modeling of a successful combination of teaching and scholarship.

STORY INTRODUCTION

Dr. Rew's love of community health nursing, with its focus on patient education, solidified her interest in nursing education. Yet, the core of her work as an educator remains centered on teaching not just nursing students, but clients everywhere. She describes her teaching as permeating everything that she does, including her research and her mentoring, both formally and informally.

EARLY INTEREST IN TEACHING

My earliest interest in teaching came from my childhood. My favorite aunt was a teacher who taught first graders how to read. She was also a Christian Scientist and since I was interested in becoming a physician, we had all these tremendous philosophical discussions about whether I should go into teaching or whether I should go into medicine. I compromised by going into nursing. When I was in my basic nursing baccalaureate program, I remember looking at all those teachers and thinking that I would rather be teaching than doing patient care. My earliest interest in teaching goes way back, but in terms of teaching nursing, my interest began with my baccalaureate program. I saw my instructors and thought that I would like to be an instructor. I started at the University of Iowa in a pre-nursing program and completed 1 year there. Then I went to Iowa State University and took a little detour. I studied modern languages for a year. Then I married my childhood sweetheart. When my husband was sent to Hawaii for 3 years as a pilot in the Navy, I decided to go back to school. By then, I decided that I would study nursing rather than modern languages because nursing had a more practical application. I completed my baccalaureate degree at the University of Hawaii and graduated 10 days before my twins were born. They are 36 years old now. One is a nurse and one is an attorney, girl and boy; the girl is the nurse.

PREPARATION FOR TEACHING

After working as a clinical nurse for 5 years I decided to go back to school for a master's degree. My husband was in an MBA program and once he finished it was my turn to go to school. While he was in school, I took a job in a community hospital as the staff development instructor. I worked with a man that was not very good at his job in staff development, but I learned a lot of things from him, including what not to do. That really piqued my interest in being an educator. I knew that education was definitely more my calling than actual clinical nursing. I was much more comfortable when I was actually teaching patients something. I learned from my colleague in staff development how to teach new teachers. That was my very early preparation for teaching. Then I got a master's degree in community health nursing.

I loved the fact that community health nursing was very focused on teaching. We had a very diverse clientele in community health. I envisioned that the perfect nursing job would be that I could teach people about their health. When I finished my master's degree, I figured that while I was going to school, I might as well just keep going on. I went immediately into the doctorate education program. I found out that I had to do 9 hours of master's level course work in education. That was at Northern Illinois University. By that time I had two little children at home and I was working part time. I completed my doctorate by the time I was 35. My doctoral focus was on counseling education; it was designed primarily for school counselors. When I went into the program, I had to meet with a panel of interviewers who got to decide whether they wanted to admit me or not. When they were finished talking with me, they called me back in and said that it sounded to them like I really should go to medical school rather than to their program. I said that I would love to go to medical school, but I had two small children and a husband who flies, I did not think I could manage medical school with those constraints. They then admitted me to the doctoral program.

I learned a lot of counseling techniques in my doctoral program. We had to have counseling ourselves and to supervise people who were counseling students. The last year I was in that program we were to do an internship that was related to what we wanted to do when we graduated. What I wanted to do actually had never been done before. I went to my committee and said that I wanted to work in a medical group. I wanted the physicians to send their patients to me for education and counseling. I found a medical group of 13 physicians who agreed to have me work with them. One of the medical physicians in this medical group was a woman internist who thought that my idea was intriguing. She said that she would love to send her patients to me for she did not have time for patient teaching and the nurses who worked with her did not have the time or expertise to do the patient teaching. I did the internship for a semester. When I finished with it, the medical group invited me to join them as they had had such good response from the patients about what I was doing. I joined them and developed a service called Patient Education and Counseling. I worked there for 3½ years before I moved to Texas to be a real educator. I then joined the faculty at University of Texas.

MENTORING FOR TEACHING

My mentors have come in different forms. There are some people that I have worked side by side with that I really admire as teachers. However, a lot of my mentoring has come from reading books by great people who taught through their writing. One person who comes to mind is Martha Rogers. I was teaching in a community college at the time her first book on nursing theory was published. I remember the discussions that I had with my colleagues about her ideas, how wild they were, and at the same time, how down to earth they were. Some of the best mentoring I received was when I got to the University of Texas and actually saw how faculty combined their research with their teaching. I also wanted to develop the ability to be personable with my students and to meet my students where they were.

Helen Erickson had a big impact on me and my teaching. She took a personal interest in me as a scholar and helped me to be a better teacher. Back to my childhood, the best mentor I ever had in teaching was my aunt, because she would teach in some of the most subtle ways. She taught mostly by example, by the way she lived her life. That made an indelible impression on me at a very young age. It was something that I never forgot; she taught me how to be kind to everybody. I grew up on a farm. I was a poor kid. Neither of my parents went to college. This aunt represented something that I did not have in my own home. Whenever she would come to visit, she would read to my brother and me. She would always bring games for us to play. She was always very organized and systematic about things. We always ended up learning something from her, even simple things like how to dress, or how to fix your hair, or how to be polite to people. Those things were part of who she was, and we wanted to be like her. In my little girl mind, I wanted to be just like her when I grew up. I would hear her tell stories about how there might be a poor child in her class who came to school on the coldest day of winter and did not have a jacket. She would go and buy a jacket. The next day when it was time for him to go home without saying anything else, she would just put the jacket on him and send him home.

My sponsor at the University of Minnesota, where I did my postdoctoral work, was a man named Michael Resnick, Director of Research in the pediatric program, and a sociologist by training. He was a mentor to me and recently wrote the foreword for my book on adolescent health. He is a magnificent teacher. He is one of the people who teaches constantly. He is an outstanding classroom teacher, as well as an everyday mentor. He would

frequently say, "Well, what do you want to do? Of course you can do that."
He constantly gave encouragement and believed in me and the other fellows in our program.

EVOLUTION AS A TEACHER

I have been around so long, I feel that I must know how to do something
right. I am able to hear a lot of myself with my students. Rather than having them see me as some "expert" on a pedestal, I try to understand them,
to find out the tools they need to be successful in their lives. The teaching
I try to do is very person-oriented, very person-centered—not so much
what I am trying to impart on them, but, "What do I know that I can share
with them, that they can take forward and make their lives better?" This belief comes from the research I am doing now with homeless adolescents. We
are doing a sexual health intervention with them. One of the basic principles I have to make certain is that the interventionists understand that they
should not go into the intervention as the expert, because they are not.
These adolescents can tell the interventionists more about life and more
about sex than they have ever dreamed of knowing. Yet they have some information that the adolescents do not have. They have to figure out how to
share that information with the adolescents in a way that is nonthreatening,
in a way that they can pick up and use to their advantage. These adolescents
are not going to come back and see the interventionists as the great guru
that saved their life. That is not what it is all about.

When I meet a student where they are and say, "Hey, what is it that you
need to move on in your life and to develop right now? What information
do I have or what experience do I have that I can share with you that will
help you go wherever it is that you want to go?" I am not at all afraid to tell
my students about all the mistakes that I made. I teach a professional writing class right now. A lot of writing for publication is about getting rejected,
and saying to them, "Guess what, so did I." I tell them what to do with re-
jection. You figure out what skills you need to improve. What other resources do I need to reach the goal that I set for myself?

FEELING COMFORTABLE AS A TEACHER

In the first 5 years that I was working in staff development in the hospital I
felt comfortable after 6 months doing what I was doing. However, when I

moved on to the junior college and had to learn to deal with a different kind of student, it took me a year to get comfortable doing that. Then, when I moved to the University of Texas and had to deal with college and university level students, and graduate students, when I had never worked with graduate students before, it took me a couple of years to be comfortable. It also depends on the topic. I have taught so many things in my career. I have taught clinical psychiatric nursing to undergraduate students. I have taught pediatric clinical to undergraduate students. I have taught community health nursing to undergraduate students. I have taught practically everything at the master's level. I have taught every core course within the doctoral program, from theory to philosophy to research methods to now a professional writing course. Each one of these teaching experiences has been a little bit different. I feel comfortable teaching anything that I feel I know fairly well—if I feel I know it well enough to write an article about it.

CHALLENGES AS A TEACHER

Facing students who you suspect are cheating in your class is a big challenge. How do you confront somebody when you think you saw him or her cheat? I do not want to believe those kinds things about my students, and yet I know it happens. It is very uncomfortable to have to confront a student about academic dishonesty. Working with a student for a long time and then realizing that they really do not have the potential to do what they want to do is really a challenge. I have faced it more than once.

EMBARRASSING TEACHING MOMENTS

I was teaching an undergraduate pediatric course. I had been teaching things about the heart for years, and I had this standard way I drew the heart with all the chambers and all the vessels coming in and out of it. I got my teaching evaluation that year and one of the students had the gall to write on there, "She doesn't even know how to draw an accurate diagram of the heart." I thought that was the craziest thing that I had ever heard and it really bothered me. It embarrassed me because I had been drawing it the same way for so many years. I went back to my books, and it was not inaccurate, but I thought that if the executives reading the evaluation would believe that for a minute, that would be embarrassing.

REWARDING ASPECTS OF TEACHING

I would say right now is the most rewarding time in my teaching career, as we are conducting this teaching intervention. My teaching is permeating everything I am doing in my research. I am not teaching a formal course this semester, but I feel like I am teaching on a daily basis. I employ at least 10 staff members for the two funded research studies I am directing. They are young people who I teach every day when I walk into my research center. We have a longitudinal study going on in the schools in the Austin area; I send at least 5 Research Assistants every day to collect data from these students. One of the things I love about working with these young people is when I say to them that I know their job is pretty well circumscribed, but we are gathering so much useful data that if they have an idea about an article they would like to write, they should let me know about it. I feel like I am helping them develop professionally and personally while doing this important job.

LEAST REWARDING ASPECTS OF TEACHING

I had to do some team teaching with new students. Each one of us was supposed to teach in our specialty area. You would come in and do your guest lectures three times and then the rest of the time you were supervising students in the clinical area. The students would rotate every 3 weeks. I did not like that because I did not get to know any one group of students very well. They were constantly changing. I think the same thing could be said of my work in staff development. We would do CPR training, emergency medical training, and teach the same thing over and over again. That is not me; I am far too creative for that. I need to have more experiential interactions with students, where I can get to know them on a one-to-one basis and help them each develop in a unique way.

MAINTAINING EXCELLENCE AS A TEACHER

I continue to learn from others, e.g., by watching other people who I know are good teachers. I try to learn something every day from books, articles, people on the radio, and lectures. I try to analyze how I can change my actions to be more like the persons that I admire. Also, I work on maintaining excellence on a daily basis as much as possible. I do a lot of brainstorming. I take a notebook with me every day and try to write things down about ideas that I have, for changes, etc.

ADVICE FOR NEW TEACHERS

Keep teaching until you become comfortable. But do not do it unless you really love teaching. Do not believe too much in your own expertise. Your job as a teacher is to help somebody learn—not to put ideas in their head, but rather to help them discover things. Two of my best teachers have been my own children. We think we will show them the world as parents, but these children show us the world. My philosophy on raising children is not that I have to give them all this stuff so that they can grow up to be competent and caring, etc. I have to make an environment that is safe enough that they can discover who they are and be who they are. In the process I am going to be treated by learning. I watch my son with my granddaughter and think of my son as an infant, and see that he is the parent of an infant. I watch him and think about what he is doing, how he is trying to teach her, and what the messages are that he is giving. It is a whole new learning experience for me because I know I will learn a whole lot about myself and the world through the eyes of my granddaughter. It is the same with students—you never know who you are going to touch with something that you do or do not do. Students will come back to me years later and say that I taught them something, and that they have never forgotten it. That is a reminder that we should be careful what we say to our students, and how we act in front of them. There is always an ethical responsibility to be attentive to what we say to students.

Even though I have never received a teaching award, it is rewarding to hear peers speak of my teaching excellence. My students at my first real teaching job at the community college said that I was "like a breath of fresh air."

CHAPTER 17

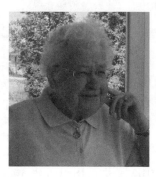

Grayce M. Sills

BACKGROUND

Dr. Grayce M. Sills is Professor Emeritus at the College of Nursing, The Ohio State University. She holds a diploma in nursing from Rockland State Hospital, a BSN from the University of Dayton, and MS and PhD degrees from The Ohio State University.

She has served as past president of the American Psychiatric Nurses Association and the American Nurses Foundation, and editor of the *Journal of the American Psychiatric Nurses Association.* She was elected a Fellow of the American Academy of Nursing and served 8 years as a member of its Governing Council. Dr. Sills is a founding editor of the *Journal of the American Psychiatric Nurses Association.*

Dr. Sills has numerous scholarly publications. Her recognitions and achievements include The Ohio State University's Distinguished Service Award and Distinguished Teacher Award, an honorary Doctor of Science degree from Indiana University, Nurse of the Year by the American Psychiatric Nurses Association, a Living Legend of the American Academy of Nursing, and the Hildegard Peplau Award from the American Nurses Association for contributions to psychiatric nursing.

STORY INTRODUCTION

Dr. Grayce Sills's dedication to nursing and the development of the practice of psychiatric nursing is best demonstrated by her belief that her greatest accomplishment is her work with graduate students. She holds that the content to be taught is derived from the student's clinical experiences and that the teacher is a consultant with the student in the learning situation.

EARLY INTEREST IN TEACHING

I first became interested in teaching when I was a freshman in high school. I grew up in a very small town and was sent from the high school over to the elementary school as a substitute teacher because they did not have regular substitute teachers. I had the little people in class, enjoyed it, and thought this is really neat. At that time, I do not think it crystallized that I wanted to be a teacher, although that experience certainly helped frame a later decision.

PREPARATION FOR TEACHING

After graduating from the diploma program at Rockland State Hospital, I received a New York State Mental Health Department tuition waiver to go to Teachers College (TC) at Columbia University to complete my degree. At TC, they thought I was a whiz-kid since I already had 2 years of college before Nursing School. I had a diploma in nursing under my belt and hit TC at the time when they were closing their baccalaureate program and beginning to offer master's programs. Mildred Montag was my advisor, and she said, "Well, you know, you're kind of an exception and we could start you in the master's program with Hildegard Peplau even though you don't have a bachelor's." So then I was working on a bachelor's and a master's which had to be interrupted after a year and a half when I returned to Ohio to help my sister and her family. I fully intended to return to TC but never did. During that year and a half, the administrators at Rockland State Hospital said that since I had 2 years of college I could now teach. So, I began teaching. I taught history of nursing, drugs and solutions, and several other courses that were divided up in small bits. I just did it without much guidance or assistance or help. I had one course in teaching at TC. It was taught by a fine professor of music by the name of James Marsell. He was more of a philosopher than an educator. Perhaps, one of the best things that happened to me was that I did not finish at TC. What I mean by that is that I didn't get caught up in that era (early 1950s) when there was not much content in nursing and so an over-focus on education. It was thought that nursing education was having all the objectives in order, and studying students instead of nursing practice. I did not get caught up in that thinking.

When it looked like it was possible, I moved to acquire the master's. At that time, there were two people at Ohio State teaching in the only graduate program in psychiatric nursing in Ohio at the time. They were not eager to have me as a student in their program. They knew I came out of an interpersonal orientation and they came out of a psychoanalytical orientation. While we were friends, it was mutually determined that it was not a good idea for me to do my graduate study with them. We decided that what might work was a graduate program in sociology, a master's in sociology where I could focus on medical sociology. If I were studying organizational sociology, I could study hospitals. If I were studying deviance, I could study mental illness. It was a matter of goodness of fit at Ohio State. At that time the psychology department was very experimental and very "rat oriented" while the sociology department had a broader orientation, they even had a family counseling program. So, it was a more favorable environment, for my work. I had a superb group of faculty—a group of university faculty who were, at that point in their careers, coming to be nationally known, and were just about to become internationally known. They were very accessible to students. All during my graduate study I went to the VA hospital in Lexington, Kentucky, as a consultant, and worked with the staff on developing their clinical skills in one-on-one groups. So, I kept my identity as a nurse alive during that period and never expected to think like a sociologist. But, to my surprise, I began to think like a sociologist. I think I still have a more sociological view of nursing, than a "nurse-ological" view of nursing.

MENTORING FOR TEACHING

And so it was a blessing that I did not finish at Teachers College and also a blessing that I had the opportunity to begin a relationship with Hilda Peplau. I had life-long mentoring from her. More important, I learned a teaching method. Her doctoral dissertation at TC was on the "Experiential Method of Teaching." In this method, the content was derived from the clinical experience. This automatically put the teacher in a different relationship with the student. You were collaborators in the process. The student was gathering the data and as teacher you were helping analyze, providing references and that kind of thing. It was clear that a teacher needed a broad theoretical background in the field in order to relate with the clinical content that was developed out of clinical practice. This method always seems to have made for a different style of teaching. It was more about being a consultant with students. Hilda always said, "One should never refer to the students as my students." She would say, "They studied with me." I try to incorporate that in my language as well. Student and teacher both learn from the clinical data at the same time. Now presumably, the teacher has more experience, or should have, by definition, a broader range and command of the literature in psychology, psychiatry, and the social sciences to help people interpret the phenomenon that they are dealing with.

EVOLUTION AS A TEACHER

When I returned to Ohio, I was helping with family problems, and decided that I would stay in Ohio for a year before returning to TC. I wanted to work in a state hospital. When I talked to the people in the State Mental Health System they said, "We would like to have you anywhere!" "Anywhere" ended up being at Dayton State Hospital where I took an administrative position that was both clinical and administrative. However, I was distressed because there were somewhere between 90 and 110 nursing students for a 3-month period who lived on the grounds. It was a 12-week experience in psychiatric nursing. I was taken by the fact that none of them ever returned as staff. So, when the faculty in charge of the program left, I said, "I want to be in charge of the program." I was piling up years in college, but still had not finished my baccalaureate. At this time in the mid to late 1950s, there was less concern about what academic credential you had. I worked on finishing the baccalaureate part time at the University of Dayton and began to work with the students who came for their psychiatric nursing experience on affiliation.

I worked with two other people teaching psychiatric nursing to the students. We taught using the clinical data that the students brought from their care of patients. Some days we would focus on anxiety, some days on depression, and some days on hallucinations. We were zooming along just fine until I had a call from one of the home schools that asked me for the course outline and objectives. They were preparing for a State Board visit. We didn't have any! We got busy and someone sat at the back of the room taking notes from the class. After each class we wrote up the objectives and the content. This experience led to my lifelong aphorism that states, "Never let an objective interfere with learning." I have seen too many examples of people getting frozen into thinking that "this is what we are to learn" and "we can not learn anything else." One must always be open to the possibilities for learning that go beyond the objectives. We got through that first round of having the State Board visit, which was an educational experience for me. Hilda always said that the word education comes from the Greek word 'educe,' which is "to be led out of" or "to bring out of." Her idea was that you educed from the clinical data, the content. She built the content of psychiatric nursing through her work with students at Teachers College. I believe the method is as valid today as it ever was. The actual acquisition of knowledge may be a little easier, because it is more structured than it was in those early years. Hilda often came in the summer and we did some summer workshops together. She kept pushing me, telling me I needed to work with graduate students, and to do that I need a master's, and probably a PhD. I felt her gentle knuckles in my ribs while at the same time was very happy at Dayton enjoying what I was doing. I enjoyed the clinical work and watching the students learn and grow. More importantly, they came back to the hospital and worked with us. The only part of work at Dayton that I did not enjoy was the supervision of the student nurses dormitory. That was not my strength because I am not good at rules and housemother kind of things. That piece of the work was not my favorite.

I had a year between the master's and the doctorate, and took a position at Ohio State teaching psychiatric nursing in the undergraduate program in the school of nursing. I think that was one of the hardest periods of teaching I ever had. I was teaching in a program that was analytically oriented and I was interpersonally oriented. It was really tough trying to keep my viewpoint and my passion about my viewpoint under control so that it was not disruptive to the students or the program. I was not very successful, but I lived through it. I told the director of the school that I did not think it was working because the people who headed the program and I were too far apart. She told me that of the most important experiences in her doctoral program was a course in which two philosophers articulated their different points of view to the students. This did not happen for me in this year of undergraduate teaching; it was most difficult.

FEELING COMFORTABLE AS A TEACHER

I think I've always felt comfortable in a classroom. It's never felt unfamiliar. I believe this has to do with the way I teach. One of my methods is to know as much about the people who are in the room with me as I can, even if it is an audience of 400. I try to find out how many of them are only children, how many of them are from large families, how many are rural, how many are urban, how many of them are diploma graduates, how many of them have "this" kind of degree, how many are married, how many are single.

Then, I can use examples, illustrations, and stories that will tie into the experiential background of the people who are in the room. This "knowing" the audience brings a level of comfort. When comfort is absent, and sometimes it is, when I have not been able to make it happen, it is dreadful; but that is a rare occurrence.

CHALLENGES AS A TEACHER

Hilda and I did a large weeklong workshop for nurses in the state of Ohio on interpersonal counseling and working with a group of very difficult patients. I had half of the students and Hilda had the other half. By the second day, there was already some mumbling in the background about some of them having the great Hilda Peplau and some of them having Mrs. Sills. There were some sessions where we had them together and as soon as Hilda got a whiff of the mumbling, she addressed it. I remember her standing in front of the group saying, "Some of you are concerned that you are getting 'less than' with Mrs. Sills than you are with me. Let me assure you, you are getting 'equal to and more than.' When they made Grayce, they broke the mold." I never will forget it. It was such an affirmation of belief in my potential and capacity. I think that is one of the most valuable things that a mentor does is to somehow signify a belief in the potential and capacity of the person. She always gave me gentle nudging about career guidance. The opportunity to work with her side by side and to debrief with her guided my learning of so many basic fundamental concepts. For example: start with people where they are, take them as far as you can, value everybody's experience. These learnings seeped into every pore. I did all the things that you do initially with a role model mentor. I tried to stand like she stood and tucked my thumb in my skirt belt the way she did. I knew that those weren't the things that did it, but, early on they were the things that gave me some kind of reassurance from time to time. For many years with Peplau, it was senior to junior mentoring. It was only in the last 20 or 25 years of her life that it was much more collegial.

EMBARRASSING TEACHING MOMENT

It was early on in my time after my PhD. Among other things, Hilda said that I really should learn about family therapy because that's the new, emerging thing. So, I went to the University of New Mexico workshops that she, Shirley Smoyak, and Bill Field were doing. When I returned to Ohio State, I took on a couple who had a baby for family therapy. I had a graduate student ask to go with me to observe. I said yes. We were in the middle of the time with the couple when the wife excused herself and went toward the kitchen. We waited, me, the student, and the husband. Five minutes, 10 minutes, 15 minutes, and finally after about 20 minutes the wife returned and said she had called suicide prevention and that now she felt better. Although this was embarrassing at the time, as I look back on it now, it is funny. But I learned from that experience, too.

REWARDING ASPECTS OF TEACHING

I think the most rewarding period is one that I call the "golden era." It was about a decade in the graduate program at Ohio State where we fashioned a new curriculum. We were able to design it around a different paradigm from traditional nursing. Most importantly we had a group of faculty who believed in it and who shared a common belief and value system. We managed to maintain that for almost a decade and it was a wonderful time. It was a time when you worked collegially with your friends and colleagues and looked for the expansive cutting edge. We were working on putting together what it really meant to think about nursing as a holistic healing profession and to have advanced clinical expertise. It was a wonderful time. The students of that era, who came through that program have gone on to do some remarkable things. They have gone on to positions of leadership, to do fine clinical work, and to do exciting and different things. I was interviewed for one of those articles that people write about you after a certain age. They asked how they would know a student of mine? I said, "I'm damned if I know. One of my students runs a quilt shop. She says that it's a place where she does therapy with older women who are depressed. These women tell her that she has saved their lives and she teaches them quilting. While quilting in groups she also does therapy. Another one is writing children's books. Another one is writing music for a Women's Barber Shop Quartet, and doing stress reduction workshops for them."

LEAST REWARDING ASPECTS OF TEACHING

I don't think there was *any* teaching experience I ever had that was *not* rewarding. I always learned from each experience. You learn how to manage difficult situations, how to convert people to your point of view without creating revolution, and how to deal with irrational authority. There were some satisfying happenings in that tough year that I taught between my master's and my PhD. Some students from that experience will tell you to this day that it was the best thing that ever happened to them. The teaching was vital. The outcomes were good, but it was a tough year.

MAINTAINING EXCELLENCE AS A TEACHER

When I hear myself getting irritated with students, that is a barometer that tells me I am too far away from practice myself. Being involved in practice gives you the humility you need to work with people who are learning from their practice. By this I mean to know how tough it really is. So this constant refreshment and reminder has been part of the key to maintaining excellence. The other key is to read widely and keep adding to your experience. You grab opportunities to increase your experiential base because the broader it is, the more you have to share with students. When I had the opportunity to go on service boards, it was an opportunity to bring something about how agencies and organizations work. This was helpful in guiding students to think through situations in which they might be working and assessing.

ADVICE FOR NEW TEACHERS

I would tell new teachers to always be open to the new and novel. Ask yourself what you can learn form this situation. Think of teaching as a gift to make a difference. What difference will this course make in the lives of the students? I think new teachers could be helped with a course in acting to help them express their ideas.

New teachers should keep in mind that they do not own the student and that outcome measures are for the short term. It is the long-term application and verification of what students have studied that makes a difference.

You are a cocreator with the students of their learning.

If your students don't believe your words they are unlikely to believe your "Power Point" presentations.

Find a mentor . . . share your struggles.

Remember that integration/synthesis occurs when experience meets information, transformed to knowledge which can then be used and shared with others. It may occur as the syllabus suggests, but also is very likely to occur months or years after the exposure to information.

CHAPTER 18

Ursula Springer

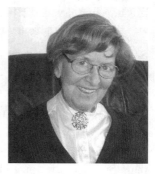

BACKGROUND

A native of Berlin, Dr. Ursula Springer studied at the Universities of Berlin, Bologna, and Munich. She received her MA degree from the University of Minnesota and her PhD from Teachers College, Columbia University. She initially pursued an academic career and, for 15 years, was Professor of Comparative and International Education at City University of New York. After her husband died in 1970, she took over his company, Springer Publishing Company. Dr. Springer is recognized for her outstanding leadership of Springer. Many Springer publications are standards for the industry, and have received numerous awards from professional organizations, including many *American Journal of Nursing* Book of the Year awards.

An early recognition bestowed on Dr. Springer was the invitation by Sigma Theta Tau International for honorary membership. In recent years, both the American Academy of Nursing and the Gerontological Society of America have named Dr. Springer as a Fellow.

STORY INTRODUCTION

Dr. Ursula Springer holds that a teacher must empathize with the learning mind and thus understand the learning mind of the student. Teaching is not telling students what they should learn but rather guiding them in how to learn. She believes that enthusiastic mentors who are master practitioners and interested in the student's learning are essential in providing an excellent education.

EARLY INTEREST IN TEACHING

I come from a family devoted to education. My mother was an excellent teacher; her interest in psychology and pedagogy motivated her to keep diaries of her 3 children's development from birth until the ages of 17, 18. Into her seventies and eighties, my mother was tutoring high-school students in French, English, and mathematics before tests and exams. My grandfather was a prestigious principal of a modern type of gymnasium (high school for boys) in Berlin. At home we often talked about school and education.

I started early showing interest in teaching: at age 6, I taught the kids of the neighborhood, so my mother gave me a portable blackboard instead of dolls. During high-school years I was constantly tutoring girls 2 or 3 years younger than I was. This provided nice pocket money and firmed up my own learning. (The Latin saying is "docendo discimus" = by teaching we learn.)

When beginning university studies in Berlin, I took up languages/literature in German, English, Italian. One year of study I spent at the University of Bologna (Italy). By now my career goal turned to teaching at university level in pedagogy (education), with emphasis on modern methods of teaching.

After 7 semesters at European universities I obtained a scholarship for a year of study at the University of Minnesota. There I learned methods and styles of education that differed from the European traditions in challenging ways. I did my master's degree and continued toward doctoral studies.

The theories of John Dewey and his contemporaries interested me and made me ever more conscious of my style and methods in teaching. In the meantime I obtained a certificate for teaching Latin, French, Italian, German, and Social Studies (from the State of Minnesota).

My practical experience began by teaching Latin in a small college-related secondary school for girls in St. Paul. My students were less interested in Latin than they were in me as their only teacher not in nun garb and German by origin. My most memorable student was Kate Millet; she often stayed at my desk after class and liked to hear about the world outside her narrow environment. She said "I want to go to New York, then to London, and then farther into the world." She did it all, became famous as an active spirit in the women's movement and the "sixties" generation. In the late 1960s, I saw her briefly at a theatre party in Greenwich Village; we recognized each other. She called out: "My Latin teacher!"

Later on, in New York, where I completed my PhD in Education at Columbia University, I became active in the newly founded Comparative Education Society. During those 3 years I taught at Pelham High School, north of New York. Besides German, I taught Social Studies for 8th and 9th grades, a very American mixture of history, geography, and basic elements of social and political science. I never had that in my own school days, but I found it interesting, and stressed geography, as this was nearly unknown to my college teachers, thus quite neglected. The school served children of privileged suburban families, thus the teaching was not problematic. One 10th grade student impressed me as remarkably knowledgeable about opera, an art form that I love. A student who sometimes scared me was one 9th grader who looked like a young gang member. In summer his shirt was open to his navel, and I saw a knife on his clothing. His family lived on "the other side" of the railroad tracks.

Those were the late 1950s, and "homeroom" was an accepted element in the schools where teachers had personal contacts with their students every morning for 20 minutes. One 9th grade girl had the misfortune to become pregnant. She asked the guidance counselor to be placed in my homeroom. It made me very proud, as it showed that the youngsters could trust me, and I supported them.

My teaching methods were based on a mix of German and American systems. The latter, of course, determined most external elements of conducting class teaching, also an emphasis on individual attention and guidance. The presentation of new materials—in American schools—was chiefly relegated to the textbooks, whereas in German schools, it is mostly the teachers' task and a professional skill. So I followed the German tradition (which is also that of John Dewey). Another German element in my teaching was a strong insistence on written corrections after tests were returned. This often met with lack of enthusiasm. But I insisted, pointing to sports where the training stresses the weaknesses, not repeating strengths all the time.

People who learn easily and who have learned a lot are usually not very good teachers, as they lack acquaintance with the slower minds. In my case my early years of experience in tutoring mediocre students gave me valuable experience in teaching slower learners. It also strengthened my patience. Usually I used praise as much as feasible, not only in general terms ("You are a good student") but more specifically: "Look how you got to solving this problem," or, "Look how you found all those facts for your report; tell us some details . . ." so students could experience recognition for their efforts.

While teaching a class, small or big, I demanded attention, absolutely. As a professor at Brooklyn College, I was given once a very large class, something like "Introduction to Education." It was for more than 150 students, in a large auditorium, where I was on stage, with a mobile microphone in my hand. I walked up and down, trying to "entertain" while teaching. Unavoidably, students in the highest rows in the back seemed bored and took out a newspaper to read. I stopped in the middle of a sentence—startling everybody—and said, "Gentlemen back there: Can't you see how I try to entertain you, mixing jokes with my teaching. And you disappoint me like that, finding the newspaper more intriguing than my presentation. What a competition! I have hurt feelings. Please!" Everyone laughed; the newspaper vanished, and I could continue my talk.

Humor is a great helping element in the classroom, but never at the expense of a person, of course. Another useful feature is the mutual help within one class. I remember how, as a young teenager, I used to help classmates with homework or test preparations. It is a matter of "chemistry" and fact. As a teacher I have occasionally put "two together." If two students (or more) are on similar levels of achievement, it is even easier.

My most embarrassing experience happened during my last year as a college professor, teaching a postgraduate course. The students were all men, about 16 of them, all majors in physical education and demonstrably not interested in any course that they needed to get their degree (either BS or MS). Several of them misbehaved, talking to neighbors, reading, or sleeping. I was more amazed than upset. This was one of the last classes I ever taught—an irony of fate to make it a total nonsuccess. When one day these nearly grown-up young men passed underpants below their tables from one to the next, laughing, I warned them that I considered this unacceptable for passing this graduate course, etc. The final test produced several failures. I gave Fs to 5 or 6 of them, preventing their finishing college for the degree. Well, I got phone calls from fathers saying "would I please change the grade . . ." "Absolutely not," was my answer. The dean called me in to request a change of grades. I explained the situation, refused to change the grades, and went home (somewhat afraid for my safety). I don't know what the final outcomes were. This was a sobering note on an otherwise quite happy and satisfying career in teaching.

I have also found that running a company requires teaching skills. I would have teaching sessions from time to time for the staff. From the beginnings of a book (acquisitions), through editing, production, marketing, selling, and shipping, I would ask individual members of departments to give prepared "introductions" to their fields of daily work. In an informal setting, the other staff members would ask questions and learn.

When I became President of Springer Publishing Company, as an educator, it was quite natural for me to take an interest in nursing education. I established the Springer Series (of books) on Nursing Education, which is still vigorous today, over 25 years later. Through publishing, I have continued to teach indirectly, by providing students and teachers with the texts they need.

CHAPTER 19

Christine A. Tanner

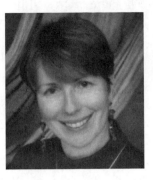

BACKGROUND

Christine Tanner earned the BSN from the University of North Colorado, MSN from the University of California, San Francisco, and the PhD from the University of Colorado at Boulder. She is the Youmann-Spaulding Distinguished Professor at the Oregon Health and Science University School of Nursing. Prior to coming to Oregon, she served as Assistant Dean for Curriculum at the University of Northern Colorado. She is a Fellow in the American Academy of Nursing and has been the recipient of numerous awards in nursing education. She teaches courses on curriculum development and evaluation, teaching strategies, and critical thinking.

Dr. Tanner's research includes accessing patient's volatility, effectiveness of nursing telephone advice, improving nurse-physician communication, and clinical decision making. She was instrumental in the founding of the Society for Research in Nursing Education.

STORY INTRODUCTION

Dr. Tanner believes that there are multiple models for curriculum, multiple pedagogical theories, and multiple philosophies that can guide the work of teaching. She is working with a statewide group of nurse educators who are redesigning nursing education by incorporating research evidence on student learning, expertise development, and clinical judgment into the curriculum. She is passionate about new and exciting ways that can transform nursing education and raise the level of nursing practice needed in today's society.

EARLY INTEREST IN TEACHING

I became interested in teaching while in my undergraduate nursing program. I had experiences with great teachers and not-so-great teachers, and really respected the fabulous teachers. I saw how much of a difference they could make for students by helping them learn complicated material. Then, when I finished my undergraduate program, I worked in the nursing intensive care unit and found myself looking for a change. I wanted a challenge and had not given much thought to being a teacher. In those first few years I really liked and enjoyed nursing, while at the same time I needed to advance myself a bit.

So, I went back to school into the master's program at the University of California, San Francisco, and began to take course work to become a clinical specialist in medical-surgical nursing. Back then, course work was also available and recommended for students to prepare in a "functional area"; I chose nursing education courses. Marlene Kramer taught the microteaching course which was just wonderful. We examined various teaching strategies, videotaped teaching sessions, and received feedback from peers about our performance. It was a wonderful way to learn and helped me to feel more comfortable with myself in a teaching role. I took a course on curriculum development from Shirley Chater and that too was a wonderful experience. When I finished the degree, I moved back to Colorado and was looking for either a clinical nurse specialist position or a teaching position. I was open to either one and quite prepared to do either one too. I ended up going back to my alma mater, the University of Northern Colorado, and began my teaching career.

Actually, I fell in love with teaching and think the most wonderful part about it is seeing students really connect and get something for the first time. It is such a reward to see students grow personally from their experience in nursing and understand that nursing is meaningful work that contributes to their own growth. As a teacher it is exciting to see students integrate their experiences, their view of themselves, and their worldview.

PREPARATION FOR TEACHING

I had good clinical expertise in nursing before I went into teaching. I felt solid as a clinician and had learned how to think things through. In my preparation we did not focus on the memorization of facts, but rather on reasoning through something by remembering discreet facts and pulling them together. I valued this approach as a student and began to do the same thing with the students I was teaching in the clinical area. A lot of my teaching practices are modeled on how I was taught. Fortunately I had a lot of good teachers who were very helpful.

I was at Northern Colorado for 2 years and decided that I really wanted to learn more about teaching and more about how people learn. I really wanted to get the PhD. I did not think about a PhD until I was in the master's program and then I was very intrigued by the idea. This was in the mid-1970s and there were few doctoral programs in nursing. I believed that I had a solid knowledge of nursing, and really wanted to advance myself in teaching. So, I went back to the University of Colorado, Boulder, for a degree in educational psychology with a minor in cognitive psychology. My research interest was in studying how nurses make decisions. I had observed in my early teaching experience that students had enormous difficulty in making sense of clinical situations. Even though they could recall factual information, they had difficulty turning that around to make good judgments about what went on in the nursing care of patients. At that time, we were using academic nursing care plans where students would write 40 or 50 pages in preparation for clinical practice. Most of what they wrote did not have very much to do with the individual patient. These plans were more or less what students could pull out of the textbook about a person having a particular kind of diagnosis. I found that there was very little connection with what the students wrote on these care plans and what they actually did in practice.

I remember one student who was in the neuro-intensive care unit and taking care of a patient who had a craniotomy. She wrote on her care plan that she would be worried about him developing diabetes incipidus because of the location of the lesion. She had a nursing concern about the potential for dehydration and was going to prevent this by was clamping the foley catheter. I was reading her care plan over coffee while the students were getting report on the unit, and I bolted up eight flights of stairs to make sure she hadn't followed through on her intervention. Of course she had not, and I asked her "What in the world were you thinking?" She said, "At 2:00 in the morning, that was the only independent nursing intervention I could come up with." This is one example of many that suggested the way we were trying to help students reason really made very little sense. I wanted to find another way of helping students to reason through nursing care situations, which started me on my research career around clinical decision making/clinical judgment.

I continue to be interested in clinical decision making to this day. I believe it is critical to look at how this research and research like it can be translated into the practices of educators. Over the last several decades, research has shown us a great deal about how people learn. If this research were used in our practice as teachers, it would truly transform nursing education.

MENTORING FOR TEACHING

I was involved in staff development at a veteran's hospital in California, and one of my colleagues, Ann Huntsman, was an incredible mentor. I got really nervous when I spoke in front of groups. She helped me to make myself feel comfortable when speaking to groups. When I started my teaching career in Colorado, the school had one of those big 1970s-style curriculum grants to revise the curriculum. Lida Thompson, who was in charge of the grant, was excellent in working with faculty who had very little teaching experience. We really worked on thinking about nursing conceptually, and then how one would help students apply the concepts clinically. She did not stand beside me and help me think about teaching, but really helped me work on conceptual thinking. Conceptual thinking is critical to teaching effectiveness. In addition, Dean Phyllis Drennan was instrumental in my pursuing doctoral study in my early career. She was a cheerleader for me who had confidence that I would make important contributions. She did everything to get me into national circles, which was extremely wonderful and helpful. Having someone give you a shot of encouragement and confidence is so important when you are taking on a new role and not sure that you can be successful in the new role.

Shirley Chater and Marlene Kramer were in some ways also my mentors. They were teachers in large classes of 40 to 50 people at UCSF. The work they did with us in the class, felt a lot like personal touch. That seemed, as I think back, to be really important, even in the large classes. They commented on the papers I wrote in positive ways.

EVOLUTION AS A TEACHER

I think the study of how people learn and how people develop expertise has really transformed my teaching in many ways. In the early 1980s, I worked with Bill Holzemer in starting the Society for Research in Nursing

Education. Through that group, we collected people who had a passion about nursing education, which at that time was starting to decline because of the national focus on clinical nursing research. We believed strongly that it was important to continue the threads of nursing education research because nobody else was going to be doing it. We did not want to lose the strength in nursing education research.

Nancy Diekelmann, Pat Moccia, David Allen, Em Bevis, and several others who were involved in the Society began to think about the kind of reform in nursing education that was necessary. Each of us in our respective institutions were finding that education had become pretty stagnant, without much movement or change. We, on the other hand, were inspired with the educational literature and our own scholarly work in nursing education and believed that we needed to really push things ahead. I can remember having this discussion about stagnation in nursing education with Pat Moccia, Pam Miraldo, and Frank Shaeffer who were with the National League of Nursing at that time. Although we had worked through some of the accreditation issues, we were trying to find a way to make accreditation more of a stimulus for change that would keep nursing education from being so stagnant. Frank Shaeffer said that we were asking for a revolution in nursing education. We all agreed that was absolutely it. And so, the mid to late 1980s movement that became known as "The Curriculum Revolution: A Mandate for Change," was birthed. Many others inspired this movement along the way: Jean Watson, Peggy Chinn, Carol Lindeman, and Joyce Murray, among others. We planned a series of conferences where we brought together people to think through what changes needed to occur and what needed to happen in order to make the changes. The major contribution of that movement was to challenge old ways of thinking, and to open up new possibilities. It seemed that nursing faculty generally were stuck in accepting the old truths about how you construct the curriculum, how you write objectives, how you teach a course by telling students what they need to know. Teachers had simply not questioned the behavioral model of teaching. The point of the revolution was to say there are multiple models for curriculum, multiple pedagogical theories, and philosophies that can guide the work of teaching.

Research on Teaching

I researched how students and practicing nurses cognitively process the making of clinical judgments and continued that work after I finished my doctoral program in 1977 and into the early 1980s. At that point Patricia Benner had started publishing work on novice to expert. I still remember after her work came out in the *American Journal of Nursing,* I called her on the phone to have a discussion, because I totally disagreed with her theoretical perspective and thought she knew nothing about cognitive theory. We ended up having a several-hour debate on the phone about the different theoretical perspectives. She introduced me to another whole way of understanding human thinking; that conversation began a happy collaboration. She and I together with Margaret Grier went public with our debate, to discuss the different theoretical perspectives about human judgment. In 1986, I took a sabbatical to work with Patricia Benner; with her I studied philosophy of science, focusing on the work of Martin Heidegger, and, of course, Bert Dreyfus. During my sabbatical we conducted some preliminary studies about expertise in making judgments. We completed a full-scale study that was finished in the early 1990s, culminating in our book, *Expertise in Nursing Practice: Caring, Clinical Judgment and Ethics,* published by Springer in 1996. My work underwent a transformation through the studies with Benner and really opened up new ways to approach expertise on how nurses go about making judgments in nursing practice.

After we finished that work, I began to look for a way to study how expertise in practice, and clinical judgment specifically, could be linked to patient outcomes, and tried to find a venue in which we might be able to demonstrate this link. One of the criticisms of our work was that, although it was wonderful descriptive work, the link to patient outcomes was missing. I took another sabbatical in 2000 and went to the Kaiser Center for Health Research here in Portland to work with Barbara Valanis, on a study on nursing telephone advice. Telephone advice nursing seemed to be an excellent venue for examining unobtrusively the practice of a nurse (in this case their interaction with a caller seeking health advice, and the nursing judgments made during the interaction), and outcomes of that interaction. We ended up doing a multisite study of nurses in the Kaiser System throughout the country, by tape recording thousands of phone calls and then analyzing the recordings for communication style and judgments. We then did follow-up recorded reviews and interviews with callers to capture outcomes of care. We had virtually no variation in caller satisfaction or in follow-through on advice. We found that having access to advice from a nurse was critically important to Kaiser health plan members, and saved callers and the plan from many needless emergency department, urgent care, and medical office visits. However, we were unable to capture a meaningful measure of clinical judgment.

FEELING COMFORTABLE AS A TEACHER

I felt comfortable within a couple of years of teaching and confident in my ability to put together a meaningful course and to interact with students in meaningful ways. However, I was anxious at the beginning of every quarter with a new class of students, and to this day it still occurs. I am hyped a bit more at the beginning of a term when I am meeting with a new group of students and laying out the plan for the term. Every teacher I know has this same experience the first day of class. It is an important point of the course where there is important interaction with students. I find that in terms of comfort as a teacher, nothing ever stays the same. I have never taught a course the same way twice. I always make major revisions from year to year in courses and maintain an open flexibility about how courses are approached. I think it is so important to observe student learning and make modifications accordingly. To walk into a classroom and do it comfortably, it always takes a lot of thought and intellectual work. I do believe teaching involves a high degree of intellectual work.

CHALLENGES AS A TEACHER

I think one of the biggest challenges was working with people who really resisted doing anything differently. Nursing education to them was just fine the way it was. That sort of rigid and conservative view of nursing education is a challenge for me. I find it extremely frustrating, because as a faculty member, you're never alone as a teacher, in the sense that your contribution to the students' education is a small part of the overall experience, and so you can only be successful to the extent that you are working with a group of confident colleagues. The biggest challenges were on those occasions where I found myself working with people who had been teaching for less than a year. While we talked about using research in nursing practice, teachers didn't seem to be interested in using education research in their teaching practice. I just do not understand this position.

I think the second challenge that has been hard to overcome is the change in the generational differences in the student population. Some people are saying that students come to us with a different mindset about education. It is a stereotype of entitlement, with a customer approach. They are buying a service and they want it delivered in the way they would like to see it. I find that this is a difficult challenge to bridge. It is a chasm between how I, the teacher, view education in nursing and the perspective of the student. It is hard for me to think my class is not the most important thing in the student's life. It continues to surprise me when a student is not engaged to learn, because they want a degree and they want to become a nurse.

I have had lots of positive challenges too. What makes the work of teaching wonderful is when you can take the challenge and pull together a team of colleagues to work out solutions.

EMBARRASSING TEACHINGS MOMENTS

I was teaching a class of about 100 students on decision making. The whole course was on decision making. I really wanted to figure out ways to have them actively engage in learning. We started out the class by gathering in the large lecture hall. I arrived at school this morning, which also happened to be the first day of our accreditation visit, and was fairly certain that the visitors would be coming to my class. I arrived at school, walked into my office, looked down at my feet and noticed that I still had my bedroom slippers on. They were the big floppy kind and I had no time to do anything different than to wear them to class. So, I used the slippers on my feet as an introduction since I was teaching about decision making and specifically about diagnostic reasoning. I had the students generate hypotheses about why I was wearing bedroom slippers. It became quite the joke. The accreditation visitors were indeed there and they did comment in the report about a faculty member appearing for her class in bedroom slippers. At the end of the quarter, the whole class of students came to class in their bedroom slippers.

REWARDING ASPECTS OF TEACHING

The most rewarding time is right now. I just moved out of administration into a distinguished professorship and have this wonderful privilege of working with a group of nurse educators in the state who are redesigning nursing education, incorporating research on learning, on development of expertise, and on clinical judgment. The most exciting work I have ever done has been working with this group of people who love nursing education. They are passionate about it, good at it, and committed to educating graduates who will be at the level of nursing practice we need today. We are working on curriculum in some very new and exciting ways. I am blessed. I also am mentoring and working with young faculty who are eager to learn the teaching role. This is the best job I have ever had and a wonderful culmination for my career. All the research I have done on clinical judgment figures prominently in our work. We have technology that helps us teach students in the way that we need to teach them. We plan to admit the first group of students in the new consortium program in 2005.

LEAST REWARDING ASPECTS OF TEACHING

I had a year with some doctoral students who were not engaged. Their attitude was that they were getting their union card. However, I think overall there was hardly ever a time when I did not feel enthusiastic and challenged by my work.

MAINTAINING EXCELLENCE AS A TEACHER

I do a variety of things to maintain excellence. I think my teaching is definitely informed by my research. That is a big part of it. I really love to engage in conversations about teaching with peers here and around the country. I think in my own day-to-day practice, I am always observing and evaluating learning. The centerpiece of my work is making sure the students are learning what they need to know and getting what they want out of their course work. I try to tap into that and then modify my courses accordingly. The continuous quality monitoring on a one-to-one basis is quite important.

I have done a great deal of consulting work about nursing education research and practice. My consulting work is as informative to me as it is to people with whom I consult. Through consulting, I have time to really talk with nursing faculty about challenges in nursing education, and to think with them about how we can resolve these long-standing issues. It is truly a gift to have time to focus on our practice as teachers, and to reflect on what works, and what does not, and how research might inform that practice.

ADVICE FOR NEW TEACHERS

New teachers should stay open to conversations with colleagues about teaching and share openly what they are doing. Try to work with others to create a climate where these conversations can happen. Lee Schulman and colleagues from the Carnegie Foundation have written about teaching as a community activity or as community property. When we share little about our teaching with others, it fails to grow, and we fail to grow. Finding opportunities to engage in conversations with colleagues and figuring a way to make it happen is really important.

I think paying attention to student learning, and not taking it personally when students do not like what you do is important. New teachers do not need to get into the position of having it be very important that students like them or that they will evaluate them well. I have found that when you are being most effective is when the students are going to be least content with the way you are approaching the teaching. I think it is important to listen with an understanding that it is not always going to be a glowing report. Some of my wonderful experiences have been when students come back years later and thank me for something that was terribly difficult for them at the time and proved to be important to their overall growth over time.

It is so easy to get mired down on the day-to-day issues, debates with faculty on curriculum, issues in clinical placements, and the faculty shortage that we are all experiencing. It is important to keep faith we can get through these times and that our aim is the education of students. This is a most important and worthwhile goal that is sometimes hard to hang on to in the day-to-day grind of it all.

I think teaching is like nursing in a lot of ways. It is as much about presence and about who you are as a person. There is no way you can separate who you are as a person from who you are as a teacher. It is really important for the teacher to know self, be well grounded, and to have a certain confidence. Teachers need to engage in reflection about their work and practice as teachers in order to grow. This deep thinking about the work of teaching, engagement in the work, and commitment to it has got to be there to be successful. There are too many teachers in the world who go in and deliver their age-old lectures, walk out, and never engage with the students. They never know the students as individuals, they lose sight of who they are as people, and do not know what their commitments are. A reward of teaching is the constant ability to grow and change as a result of interaction with people. It is a strong belief of mine that teachers should know self as a person and know the influence a teacher can have on people's lives. Once a teacher is clear about self as a person, and holds an openness and recognition of the pace of change in higher education and health care, then one can look for opportunities to mold and educate students.

CHAPTER 20

Kimberly Adams Tufts

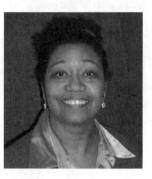

BACKGROUND

Kimberly Adams Tufts earned the BSN at The Ohio State University, and MSN and ND from Case Western Reserve University. She is an Associate Professor at Old Dominion University and is a Fellow in the American Academy of Nursing. She has been active in the area of health care policy through teaching the subject to nursing students and influencing health policy at the state level.

Dr. Tufts's research focus is HIV prevention with adolescent populations. Her school-based approach aims at advocacy activities essential to promoting the HIV/AIDS prevention and treatment agenda and to alleviating HIV transmission globally. She has lived and worked in Zimbabwe as a Visiting Lecturer in the Department of Nursing Science at the University of Zimbabwe.

STORY INTRODUCTION

Upon completion of her doctoral program, Dr. Tufts went into full-time teaching. Because the preparation in her master's and doctoral program was aimed at clinical practice, she experienced herself as underprepared for the teaching role. In order to remedy the situation, she searched out courses on how to approach the teaching of adults. Her teaching practices have evolved from a charismatic demonstrator approach into a student-centered partnership approach. She views herself as a lifelong learner who loves teaching and believes teaching is a valuable endeavor.

EARLY INTEREST IN TEACHING

Very early in my life while in high school, I had an after-school job teaching reading for 2 hours a day, 5 days a week, in a church-based enrichment center. So, I thought to myself that I liked doing this. However when I thought about a career, I thought of nursing, and at that time, I did not associate teaching with nursing. My thoughts were that I was going to college to get an education because that is what my family expected, even though they did not like nursing as a choice. So I told them, "I am going to college to be a nurse," and they accepted that. My early interest was to be a great clinician.

PREPARATION FOR TEACHING

I was prepared for teaching in an informal way. At the time I attended the graduate program at the master's level, they had taken away functional roles. I chose the clinical track and did not get a lot of formal instruction in teaching. However, I observed those who I thought were very good teachers, and took two Professional Development courses on teaching/learning. I was also a teaching assistant for one semester, completed my master's in perinatal nursing, and went on to complete a certificate program to become a nurse practitioner. I practiced 3 to 4 years in advanced practice and participated with students as a clinical preceptor. When the students were in the setting, I knew I had to approach the preceptorship in a formalized way. On the days I had students, I would rearrange my schedule to see fewer patients, which was not popular with administration. I thought there was a way to go about teaching so that the student had the structured learning experiences that were needed to be a good clinician. I taught the students in a structured stepwise fashion and got to be popular as a preceptor. Everybody wanted me to take their students.

The other thing was that people would invite me do guest lectures. I lectured on women's health and principles of community health. In my community work, I was asked to write a prenatal community outreach curriculum for a federal grant. So, I spent a lot of time reading and studying how to set up a curriculum and thinking about training the trainers. That program was federally funded and very successful. That was almost 15 years ago, when I had been out of graduate school for about 2 years.

Then, I went back for doctoral studies and after graduation thought to myself that I should teach. When I went into full-time teaching in 1996, I did not believe I was well prepared. Even though I had been a preceptor, worked on the community teaching project, and been a guest lecturer, I wondered how was I going to be responsible for complete courses by myself. So, I began to attend the University Center for Innovation In Teaching and Education (UCITE). I attended most of their sessions over a 2-year period and learned unbelievable things about pedagogy, although I prefer the term "androgyny" because, even if we teach at the undergraduate level, we are teaching young adults or adults. I teach at the graduate level so I have always been teaching adults. The root word for pedagogy is child and for androgyny, the root word is adult. I read the work of Malcom Knowles, who focuses on adult learning. Through reading his work, I began to see the difference and importance in thinking about educating adult learners instead of using the pedagogical approach. I learned about the characteristics of adult learners and how to approach teaching adults.

MENTORING FOR TEACHING

Most of the mentoring I had was informal. I would actually go to courses and sit in on courses that were being taught. When I began to teach policy, I went to the person who taught it for the doctoral program and asked if I could sit through her course. I got a lot out of that experience by observing which techniques worked and which ones did not seem to work. One of the deans at my school would give me informal tips. I remember once she asked me why my examination was so long. She told me that I needed to think about what the purpose of the examination was, and why I needed so many questions. Hearing things like that from someone who was a role model for me was helpful. I was a graduate assistant for Dr. Wilma Phipps and would get caught up in reading her materials on teaching-learning when I was suppose to be filing things.

EVOLUTION AS A TEACHER

I moved from being a "charismatic demonstrator." I learned about this concept at UCITE's end of the year spring celebration, where they brought in well known educational theorists to give a lecture. This person was from a small school in Wisconsin; he used to teach at Columbia, but left so he could focus on teaching. He said that most teachers are "charismatic demonstrators," exhibiting by your manner that you know the material. We are the experts and we demonstrate our expertise to students through our lectures; however, this is not teaching students. We know the material very well and are able to demonstrate the material, and if you are charismatic, students may learn because they are amazed as they watch you in action. They think look at this person, I would love to be like her, and so I am going to emulate her. I realized this in my first year of teaching when I won the teaching award. I continued to go to UCITE to learn in a more formal and structured way. I would read about principles of teaching-learning and started to look into and study constructivism. I just began to build my repertoire of how and what I should do and be as a teacher. My goal is that students learn basic and broad principles and that I teach them in such a way that they learn them so that they can apply them in many situations. From the very first moment I have contact with students, whether it's online via email, and especially the very first day of class, I make it known to the students that each student, wherever they are coming from and whatever their level of experience in this particular area, each and every student has something to contribute and is bringing something valued to the table. I may spend, in a 6-day course, 2–3 hours establishing this initial contact with the students. I do it by asking them certain things about themselves and find ways to acknowledge their contribution right then. For example, several weeks ago, I had 23 students in a rather large doctoral seminar and it took me 6 hours to do the introductions. I did not see it as wasted time, because what I did throughout the day was to integrate the principles of the course into our discussion. So, they immediately began to hear the new language and become invested in the course.

FEELING COMFORTABLE AS A TEACHER

I think that it took me probably about 3 years to feel comfortable with didactic teaching. This was after I finished my formal education and had attended UCITE for a year or 2.

CHALLENGES AS A TEACHER

I have been challenged by the expectations, teaching beliefs, or philosophies of some of my colleagues. What I mean is that sometimes I have thought that it was best to teach a subject in a certain way, or maybe that examinations were not needed and papers would be more important in this particular course. Some of my colleagues believed we should teach the way we were taught, and since most of us graduated from the same graduate program we used the same 26-page midterm examinations that we had taken. I thought this practice was not very productive. I did not think that this testing met our purposes. I wanted to do away with the test. In fact, before two new colleagues joined me in teaching midwifery and women's health to students, I had done away with it, but they insisted that we bring it back. It was thought that the students were not being prepared correctly because the test was not a part of the course. That was really a challenge.

My other challenge has been that I have had to learn that students come to me at different levels; some students are abstract thinkers, and some are still concrete thinkers despite being graduate students. So, the challenge for me has been how to work with each student at their level and still have them develop and grow. This has been quite a challenge.

EMBARRASSING TEACHING MOMENTS

Early on in my teaching career, probably about the second year, I taught a large group of students and I was teaching women's health. I had a student who would ask what I considered to be very concrete and not very intelligent questions. So, I would walk the room a lot using that "charismatic demonstration," turn around and answer this student with an unbelievably expert answer. On the second night I went home, and I thought about it. I thought the way I was responding to the student, even though I never said it in words, but conveying it in my manner, told her that she was dumb. The next day before the class, I told her that I had something to say to her. In front of the entire 28 students, I said, "This is what I have been doing, and it is not correct. It is demeaning, so I am apologizing to you in front of the class." It was a tough moment. The student needed to have the opportunity to develop and learn just like everyone else. I got through this and it made me a better teacher.

REWARDING ASPECTS OF TEACHING

The last 3 or 4 years have been rewarding because I am teaching subject matter that can be taught from a principle-based approach. I have been teaching doctoral students and include a course that is interdisciplinary. I love history and the law and this is what I have been teaching in the interdisciplinary course, primarily to law students. Both groups of students are highly motivated. It is because these students are self-selected. They want to be there. They want to learn the material. Many times they don't know anything about the subject matter, and the growth I see makes me feel wonderful as a teacher.

LEAST REWARDING ASPECTS OF TEACHING

The least rewarding period was when I was primarily responsible for teaching women's health to three different types of students. The advanced practice students, just like beginning undergraduate students, are very anxious and starved for the most minute details about diagnoses, tests, and medications. Given my teaching philosophy and my perspective, I am not doing them any favors by providing them minute details because the details change. When the students are anxious then I am anxious too. It does not add up to the greatest picture. However, after doing it for a year or 2, I began to relax.

I think I just entered another time in my teaching career that will be, at the least, very challenging. I am going to be teaching subjects I have never taught. I have confidence about working through the knowledge piece. However, I am going to have to learn new delivery methods. The school where I will be teaching this semester uses distance education. I am used to seminar techniques. In this new course, I will lecture via television and then have contact with the students via computer. It is going to take me some time to begin to feel comfortable, as there is going to be a rather large learning curve.

MAINTAINING EXCELLENCE AS A TEACHER

I maintain excellence by continuing to learn teaching-learning theory with the new knowledge, keeping up to date with the knowledge, and continuing to learn from the students. Teaching is not a stagnant process. I am a lifelong learner of how to teach. This year, I completed a certificate in distance education by taking four courses via computer.

ADVICE FOR NEW TEACHERS

The first thing to remember is that teacher/learner is a partnership. New teachers should not be expected to know everything about the subject matter, nor about teaching methods. So new teachers owe it to themselves as well as to their students to formally learn about teaching, whether it is through taking courses, accessing on-line resources, or choosing a mentor and working with that mentor.

I love teaching. I absolutely love it! I think that in order to be good at it, you have to see it as a valuable endeavor.

CHAPTER 21

Suzanne Van Ort

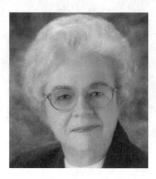

BACKGROUND

Dr. Suzanne Van Ort received a bachelor's degree from the University of Arizona, a master's degree in nursing from the University of California Los Angeles, and a PhD in education from the University of Arizona. She served the College of Nursing at the University of Arizona first as a member of the faculty and then as Dean.

She is a Fellow in the American Academy of Nursing and a Fellow in the Great Britain Royal Society of Health. Dr. Van Ort has received a number of honors and awards in nursing, including the Sigma Theta Tau Elizabeth Russell Belford Founder's Award for Excellence in Nursing Education. In honor of her contributions to nursing education, her colleagues at the University of Arizona established the Suzanne Van Ort Peer Teaching Award at the College of Nursing, University of Arizona.

Dr. Van Ort's publications are centered on the scholarship of teaching, with particular attention to baccalaureate and higher degree education in nursing. In addition, she has presented a number of scholarly papers and workshops on nursing education both nationally and internationally.

INTRODUCTION TO STORY

Dr. Van Ort's story is one of connecting to her students, as she believes that this has been one of her greatest joys in a long career of teaching. While she remained based at the University of Arizona for the majority of her long service in nursing education, her influence extends throughout the U.S. and beyond as she served as faculty and mentor of hundreds of students over her years as a nurse educator.

EARLY INTEREST IN TEACHING

I was interested in teaching and in nursing from the time I was a young person. I come from a family that has a value for learning. I remember both my mother and father encouraging teaching and learning from the time I was a young child. Our dinner conversations included, "Well, let's look that up in the dictionary," or, "Let's go find that out." It was a love of learning and imparting of that learning that began with my family. I attended a baccalaureate program in the late 1950s that was in the School of Nursing in the College of Liberal Arts. There was a focus on learning the liberal arts and sciences as a foundation for nursing. In this program I experienced good teaching and an early interest in teaching.

In the baccalaureate program I was teaching patients and learning from some expert teachers. I entered the Navy Nurse Corps after graduating from the baccalaureate program and had the opportunity to teach hospital corpsmen, which I enjoyed. Again, that reinforced an interest in teaching.

PREPARATION FOR TEACHING

I had the good fortune to go to UCLA for my master's degree in the era of Dean Lulu Wolf Hassenplug. Dean Hassenplug imparted the importance of nursing education and good teaching. So that, again, reinforced my interest. These experiences set the groundwork for more formal emphasis on teaching and on the nurse educator role.

I was in the right place at the right time for entering a PhD program in higher education with a minor in nursing. I was the first graduate in higher education from the University of Arizona and was privileged to learn from experts in higher education who were brought in as the program was evolving. I had done a number of projects on effective teaching and the doctoral program really melded my knowledge and preparation as a teacher. My dissertation was on curriculum in state colleges and universities. I focused on the history and evolution of curriculum in selected state colleges and universities around the country to track some of the trends and changes as curricula evolved. My dissertation director was Dr. Fred Harcleroad who came to the University of Arizona to begin the higher education doctoral program. My dissertation evolved from my mentor relationship with him and his interest in curriculum.

MENTORING FOR TEACHING

I was mentored in a variety of informal ways prior to the days of formal mentorship plans. As I reflect on mentoring experiences, they were with people from whom I learned the value of teaching and teaching expertise. My informal mentoring started in the baccalaureate program with Dean Pearl Parvin Coulter and Dr. Gladys Sorensen. They valued nursing education and believed faculty could and should be good teachers. Later in my master's and doctoral programs, I was fortunate to have faculty who worked with me in terms of presenting and teaching. I had a number of informal mentors and I have learned from many colleagues over the years.

EVOLUTION OF TEACHING

Initially, as a new nurse educator, I was focused primarily on covering the content and teaching what needed to be taught in the baccalaureate program. However, my teaching evolved and the focus swung to a balance of covering the content with uncovering knowledge, and discovery. This balancing was part of the evolution as I grew to value and be committed to uncovering knowledge, and to balance uncovering with covering the content. It is a different way of looking at content expertise when you also focus on what can be uncovered. Uncovering means providing the opportunity to learn new things. Part of the evolution in my teaching expertise has been an increase in creativity, focusing more on providing the opportunity for students to learn and the incentive to learn new things, all in the context of what needs to be covered. There is a focus on opening doors to discovering new knowledge or new ways of looking at knowledge. This evolution occurred with a foundation in teaching that grew over time. When you learn with the students, the excitement comes in the discovery, as well as in the covering of what needs to be taught.

FEELING COMFORTABLE AS A TEACHER

I have experienced different comfort levels at different points in my career. Two or 3 years after I began teaching baccalaureate students I felt comfortable. Then when I moved into teaching master's students there was initial stress associated with changing levels. The same is true when moving into teaching doctoral students. Feeling comfortable does not happen at one point in time when one says, "Ah ha, I'm comfortable as a teacher." Different levels of comfort come with different types of students and learning situations.

CHALLENGES AS A TEACHER

I have experienced a number of challenges. Two sets of challenges occurred periodically, however, not at the same time. The first challenge was the complexity of a faculty role. It is one thing to say that teaching is important, but in the academic environment, teaching, research, service, and practice are all important. So, the challenge is how to balance becoming an effective teacher along with being a researcher, being committed to community and professional service, and being committed to practice. Although I have never been in a formal faculty practice role, the complexity of that role seems a challenge comparable to that of teaching. The faculty role is a significant challenge that changes over time as one works on being an effective teacher along with balancing other aspects of the faculty role.

One of the things that helped me was setting goals for a given period of time. In other words, there are different expectations for a nontenured assistant professor moving forward to associate professor with tenure, than there are for an associate professor with tenure moving toward professor. So, there are some givens, in terms of time periods and goals, that are set by the system. There is also the need to continue your growth as a teacher and evaluate yourself in line with becoming a researcher. I was fortunate that I was in an academic environment, a research institution, so that research was important and the support system for research was in place. If you have a grant, then your teaching continues, yet your focus for a period of time also needs to be on research productivity. It is a challenge to balance those two aspects of the faculty role.

The second challenge is probably less prevalent now than it was in my career or generation. In my career, a higher education doctorate was often less valued than doctoral degrees in other disciplines. It was a challenge, in one sense, to prove your worth, and in another sense to share a value for higher education. I was educated in the era of the nurse scientist program, where nurses were graduating with degrees in the disciplines of anthropology, sociology, physiology, and psychology. I began as a nurse scientist in physiology and changed to higher education because of a health issue. I think those of us who had a degree in higher education with a minor in nursing needed to continuously try and over-achieve to show that we could participate actively in the discipline and science of nursing. I don't know if this continues to be a challenge, because we have more prepared nurse scientists in nursing at the doctoral level. It interests me now, to sit back and smile at the rebirth of commitment to the preparation of nurse educators.

EMBARRASSING TEACHING MOMENTS

I cannot think of any embarrassing or funny teaching moments to share.

REWARDING ASPECTS OF TEACHING

I have had an exciting career and my enthusiasm continues. The most rewarding period was when I was teaching master's students in nursing education while at the same time teaching baccalaureate students issues and research. I was dealing with two different sets of learning needs that really challenged my expertise to learn with the students. It was fascinating as a teacher to think about how to plan learning experiences for both groups of students. I thoroughly enjoyed it.

For me, the satisfaction is in learning with students and believing that you might make a difference in students' lives, who then might impart that to others. That is the satisfaction of teaching. I am so blessed that I have been able to connect with students.

LEAST REWARDING ASPECTS OF TEACHING

The least rewarding period occurred because of time issues when I was in administration for a long period of time. The combining of administration with teaching, a choice I made, was a challenge. As an administrator I chose to continue to teach because I believe that is where administration comes alive for students. Combining teaching and continuing to be effective while being a full-time administrator was probably least rewarding, because it could have been two 100% efforts. I was committed to being an effective teacher, but at the same time, had other pulls on my time. However, I believe it was a right choice. One of the dangers in administration is that one becomes too removed from the actual learning life. If administrators become that removed, then they may not value and appreciate the concerns of faculty and students. I know it is not intentional, but it can be a system problem. When an administrator, be it Associate Dean or Dean, becomes consumed with the administrator role, then the teaching/learning role can be far removed. I always was committed to both roles. I had the privilege of serving in two deanships and in both was committed to continuing to teach. I think it made me a much better administrator because I was sensitive to the students and faculty, and the issues they had about the learning environment. To this day I am very committed to the idea that administrators need to teach.

MAINTAINING EXCELLENCE AS A TEACHER

First of all, certainly knowledge of the literature is important. You need to be an avid reader and be computer literate in order to maintain excellence. It is important to stay current not only in the substantive field, but also in higher education and teaching. I continue to inquire about what is new at professional meetings and I continue learning from colleagues. I have always valued colleagues and the ability to learn with them. I believe one gains a tremendous amount of learning from others. I can remember when computers came in and computer assisted instruction was brand new. Some of us said, "I don't know about that." I had the good fortune to work with a colleague who said, "Well, let's write one!" From that angle, if you can write a computer-assisted instruction and use the method, then you can learn it and grow from the experience.

ADVICE FOR NEW TEACHERS

For me, it is exciting to consider the impact on a new generation of educators. My advice is to be enthusiastic, because you need to impart enthusiasm. Be prepared. That is, know what you're teaching and how you are going to teach, to achieve the outcomes you expect. Probably most important is being open to learning. Listen to the students. Learn with the students. I have a description of what it is to an effective teacher that I always carried with me and shared with students when I taught the nurse educator courses. Even though it is old, it is still good. The description of an effective teacher is giving the opportunity to learn, improving the ability to learn, and improving the incentive to learn. Those are three qualities of an effective teacher that could help a new nurse educator. Teaching is more than covering the content. Teaching is opening doors, listening to students, learning with students, and being open to and excited about teaching and learning.

CHAPTER 22

May L. Wykle

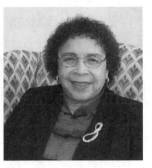

BACKGROUND

May L. Wykle is Dean and Florence Cellar Professor of Nursing at the Frances Payne Bolton School of Nursing at Case Western Reserve University. Dr. Wykle graduated from the Martins Ferry Hospital School of Nursing, and earned a BSN in nursing, an MSN in psychiatric nursing, and a PhD in education from Case Western Reserve University. She is a fellow in the American Academy of Nursing and the Gerontological Society of America. She is the past president of Sigma Theta Tau International (STTI).

She has initiated educational programs internationally and served as visiting professor at the University of Zimbabwe. Dr. Wykle has received numerous honors and awards, including the Gerontological Nursing Research Award from the Gerontological Society of America and Outstanding Researcher, State of Ohio, by the Ohio Research Council on Aging. She was the recipient of the Lifetime Achievement Award from the National Black Nurses Association, and received the STTI Elizabeth Russell Belford Founder's Award for Excellence in Nursing Education. She has published extensively, including coediting eight books, one focused on student development in nursing education.

STORY INTRODUCTION

Dr. Wykle has had a wealth of experiences in psychiatric and geriatric nursing, all of which have shaped her teaching expertise. She began her contributions to the scholarship of nursing education early in her nursing career, coauthoring a text with colleagues in the School of Education. She is well known by her students and colleagues for her humor in the classroom, and for her gift of using many life associations and experiences to emphasize opportunities.

EARLY INTEREST IN TEACHING

For several years I was a head nurse in a psychiatric institute and one of the areas that I really liked was teaching the nursing assistants. They had a huge responsibility for pouring medicines and doing assessments of patients without really having the background to do these tasks. So we began to teach them what they needed to know. At that same time, I had the experience of teaching nursing students who came to the units. In those days it was the head nurse who did the clinical teaching. We not only made the assignments and provided supervision, but also had the students for pre- and post-conferences. I really thought teaching was a neat thing to do, so I decided that I should go back to school.

PREPARATION FOR TEACHING

I received some formal preparation as part of my master's program in psychiatric nursing. Then, later on, after teaching for several years at the university level, I returned to school for a PhD in Higher Education. That opened up a whole new world; I learned much more about theories of learning, how students learn and how teachers teach. It was exciting to me to learn so much more about the classroom, and find out that as much as I wanted to teach and have students progress, learning depended on the student's readiness to learn and change. My formal preparation gave me a better idea of what you do so that students are more interested and eager to learn, rather than focusing on how well you prepare for class. I discovered different ways to learn; e.g., providing visual input at the same time as auditory input. I became aware that students do well teaching each other. When they are responsible for a class it helps them gain more knowledge about the subject. Thus, I found that seminars were most conducive to learning, particularly for graduate students.

MENTORING FOR TEACHING

At Cleveland Psychiatric Institute (CPI), I was mentored by Helen Kreigh, the Director of Nursing Education. She was taught by Dorothy Mereness and had a bachelor's degree in nursing education. I remember her saying that she had prepared a teaching outline and had presented it to Mereness for evaluation. At the end of her presentation, Mereness said, "Well, what do you think about what you have done?" Helen said, "Well, I think it is OK; but, I know I can do better." Therefore she passed that course with flying colors because Mereness said that you are always becoming, and, as a good teacher, you are never satisfied with your end product. You want to go further and achieve more, challenging both students and yourself as the teacher.

EVOLUTION AS A TEACHER

While working at CPI, I attended Case Western Reserve University and received a bachelor's degree in nursing. I really enjoyed the classes I was taking and I liked the way the teachers taught their courses. So, I enrolled in school full time and was offered a position at CPI as an Instructor of Nursing. At that time, we had 11 affiliating schools of nursing; it was a wonderful opportunity for teaching. I moved from being an Instructor to being Director of Nursing Education at CPI. It was a whole new experience for me because I had responsibility for all education programs. Every time a school was visited by the State Board of Nursing or the National League for Nursing, I had to participate. I learned quite a bit about teaching and evaluation. We had students for 3 months at a time for their psychiatric nursing experience and you had time for clinical supervision as well as the didactic teaching. There were never too many instructors—so, as Director, I did a lot of the teaching. That is how I really started my teaching career, and I thought, "I like teaching so well, I need to go back to school to improve my skills." So, I went back to get a master's degree in psychiatric mental nursing at Case on government stipend. Part of the psychiatric program at that time focused on the educative process; part of the course work was focused on application. As graduate students participating in seminars we were responsible for teaching the group classes. We spent time learning how to teach patients, following the model of Hildegard Peplau, who said that the road to mental heath was an educative process. Peplau's philosophy of psychiatric nursing fits well with the nursing model of relationship nursing.

I have always believed that teachers ought to strive to teach less so that students could learn more. It took a while for me to develop that belief over time because in the very beginning I was so oriented to teaching using a lecture format. Yet, the interactive pre- and post-conferences and seminars were so much better and I was more comfortable with students.

Another way my teaching style evolved was through teaching patients. I did some part-time work at City Hospital and did a lot of patient teaching to prepare them for surgery and discharge. Thus, I have always been involved in teaching, both formally and informally.

FEELING COMFORTABLE AS A TEACHER

I was comfortable as a teacher when I was at CPI. I think I felt comfortable because teaching was something that was expected; it was an expectation of the position. We had 11 schools of nursing so that meant having a lot of students in class. I was able to put it all together during the CPI experience: the didactic, the clinical teaching, and the integration of the two. I would say it took me about 6 months of teaching before I felt comfortable. I think part of that was because I had already had experience informally teaching patients and nursing assistants. I was always very comfortable teaching nursing assistants because I was very comfortable with the content and understood their need. They were always very eager to learn more.

I believe that for teachers the enthusiasm of the students is important. If you teach students who are enthusiastic, then you feel that you are a better teacher and enjoy the experience. I learned early in my teaching career to encourage students to ask questions. Sometimes they were reluctant to talk and to ask questions. I use to say to students, "He who asks a question is a fool for 5 minutes; but, he who does not ask could be a fool for the rest of his/her life." Encouraging students to question is a critical part of the teaching/learning exchange.

Another important factor is that I like teaching and I believe that it makes a difference. I love to lecture and I use a lot of parables and stories in my presentations. I often tell people that I am a storyteller. I think that the most important part of my preparation for classes was to be able to give examples demonstrated through parables. I have learned a lot from Gerald Kaplan, because he teaches you to understand students, and to understand your own insights about students and their ability. I love his use of the term "theme interference." He believed that sometimes the attitudes or the stereotypes that the teacher had toward the students got in the way of them being able to develop an effective teacher-student relationship.

CHALLENGES AS A TEACHER

I had some challenges, first of all, being an African American teacher when the majority of the students were not African American. I grew up in the era when bias was legal and cultural differences were exaggerated. Trying to develop cultural competence among students was a challenge. They did not call it cultural competence in those days, but it was important to help students understand the stereotypes that they had, and to be able to work with different groups of patients and staff. It was particularly important for students to understand the relationship between culture and illnesses and its effect on health promotion.

It helped me to work in a psychiatric setting, because it gave me a better appreciation for mental illness, and to understand that behavior was a question of the degree of illness. Through education, I was able to help students become less biased toward the patients. Sometimes we neglect this aspect even today; we operate on the assumption that students ought to automatically like everybody that they are working with; instead, when they do not, we need to help them to understand the importance of this.

Some of my most difficult times in teaching occurred when I tried to bring people together to learn—faculty, staff, and students. One of the skills that helped me was my knowledge of group process. It helped to bring people together and talk about a problem: What we need to discuss is in the middle of the table, let us go around and have everyone express their view on the problem. It takes the emphasis away from individual stereotypes and personal views of the situation. The other piece that is so important in teaching is being able to give feedback and do it in a structured way, and in the classroom as well. For example, in doing seminars I believe that at the end of the seminar sessions you have to be able to process the learning and have students begin to evaluate each other and be able to say, "Well, you did not do as well today as you usually do." Or, "I did not understand what you had to say." Or, "That was a really good way you led that discussion." We do not praise as much as we could. We can do that even in classroom settings. It might help students a lot more if we were to process: "OK, what was great about the class and what was not?" This evaluation process could supplement the course evaluations, which are often at the end of the course when students cannot always remember the process that occurred.

EMBARRASSING TEACHING MOMENTS

I was in a seminar once with students and they were reporting and I was absolutely exhausted. I sat in the front and closed my eyes from time to time. One of the students then asked some pointed questions because she thought I was asleep. And I was; I had nodded off, but was still able to answer the question.

I have had many embarrassing moments while being taught as a nursing student because I went to a diploma school that was very structured; you had to have the procedures down pat. Students had to go over clinical procedures time and time again, with supervision and plenty of anxiety. When I became a teacher, I was exactly the opposite because I thought the most important consideration was to keep the students' anxiety down. I have learned in teaching that humor is important and relieves tension. I tell stories that demonstrate what it is that the students need to know. This reduces the students' anxiety so that they are able to learn.

REWARDING ASPECTS OF TEACHING

My early days as a teacher were important because it helped make my decision to go back to school to learn more and get a master's degree. I thought that there were skills that I needed to know in order to be a better teacher. It was rewarding to discover that there was much to learn about teaching.

I enjoyed teaching the students from the 11 schools affiliated with CPI. To me it was rewarding because I could see the change in the students over the 3-month period of affiliation. It was possible to develop even better teacher–student relationships over the 3 month period. I still maintain that, for nursing students, you have to model that student–teacher relationship so that they can learn how to develop therapeutic nurse-patient relationships. That is why I believe it is so important that the student experiences the teacher as a person. I also believe in letting students participate in designing their own program of learning. It took a while for me to learn this because in the early days, I was so used to lecturing. Also, it is important to understand what students themselves bring to the learning experiences. Not only should I, as the teacher, bring examples to the classroom, but I should expect students to bring examples as well.

LEAST REWARDING ASPECTS OF TEACHING

My least rewarding teaching experience was when I first started as a faculty member at Frances Payne Bolton School of Nursing. I was not assigned to any formal courses for teaching, which I was really eager to do. Rather, I was asked to be a psychiatric nursing integrator, which meant that I met with hospital unit nurses to help them understand the emotional needs of patients to whom they were assigned. I went to maternity and pediatric units, medical and surgical units and any place else in the hospital where a need was identified. I was not comfortable with this role because the meetings were scheduled on an as-needed basis. They would call me and I would have to come to the units quickly and consult about a particular illness or problem situation. I did not always have any time to prepare for the teaching that I was asked to do. And I got lots of calls. Sometimes I would get 50 to 60 calls within a month. Finally the light came on for me and I understood that I needed to have more control over what was needed, rather than running back and forth from the school to the hospital on call. I decided to set up regular unit appointments to meet with the nurses and discuss problems that they were experiencing with patients. I organized seminars for them, usually around themes that would be common for the types of patients on their units. For example, I would teach them about pain management and help them understand that pain was a real problem for the patient. I used a problem presentation approach, letting them discuss the case, and then helping them identify the key components of best nursing care for the patients. As a group then, they were able to solve the problem and to gain insight into their own views about patients. Consultation became a rewarding experience and the emergency calls were reduced. I developed a positive teaching relationship with the nurses on the unit. I arranged to go to units at scheduled times. Sometimes I would go every week, or every 2 weeks. I was able to use those clinical experiences in my work with faculty and students at the school of nursing. I would provide consultation to the faculty and students during unit post-conferences.

ADVICE FOR NEW TEACHERS

My advice to new teachers is first of all, deal with their own anxiety around teaching and realize that they don't have to be so structured or that they need to have all the answers. Many new teachers will say, "OK, this is all I am going to teach," and are rigid about the course content. I believe that teaching ought to always be fun, and that when people enjoy, they learn. That is why I believe the use of humor is important for beginning teachers and they should be taught to lighten up.

There is a new two-volume book on teaching that I would recommend for educators. It is titled *Teaching Nursing: The Art and Science,* by Linda Caputi, EdD, RN, and Lynn Engelmann, EdD, RN (published by the College of DuPage Press, 2004). Also I would recommend the book that I wrote many years ago on teaching; it was coauthored with Litwak and

Sakata. In that book we discussed concerns that students have around the learning experience. Teaching to me is helping students meet their developmental needs. I believe that teachers need to know where students are in terms of their development, and that student development is a critical part of any teaching-learning process. If you can assess where students are and where you want them to be, you can be a much better teacher.

CHAPTER 23

Joyce J. Fitzpatrick

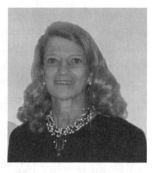

THE EARLY YEARS:
INITIAL INTEREST IN TEACHING

As an undergraduate student in the School of Nursing at Georgetown University, I decided to dedicate my future work to improving nursing education. One of the primary reasons was the fact that I admired the faculty who taught in the School of Nursing, for their dedication to what they were doing. They were committed to developing nursing as a profession and encouraged us as undergraduates to pursue graduate study in nursing. There was a high energy level among the faculty and a major emphasis on advanced education. At the same time, I felt that there was great potential for growth within the discipline of nursing. I did not believe that I was as intellectually challenged as I should have been as an undergraduate student at a major university. I viewed my colleagues in other disciplines as having more scholarly debates, more intellectual discussions about broad social and political issues, compared to those of us studying in the School of Nursing. I was disappointed that so much of the focus of nursing education was on memorization and recall, and too little was on challenging existing knowledge. I vowed to make a difference in nursing education nationally (for at that time there was little focus on global health or nursing) and made a commitment to obtain the highest level of education possible in nursing. I knew then that I would become a teacher and a leader in academic nursing.

FORMAL AND INFORMAL INFLUENCES: EDUCATION AND MENTORS

Immediately following graduation from Georgetown, I entered a master's degree program in nursing, and pursued a clinical focus in psychiatric mental health nursing with a minor focus on nursing education. I had a significant introduction to educational philosophies during this graduate program, and was introduced to the current issues and debates in nursing education nationally, including the entry level debate; the disciplinary content focus on care, cure, or coordination; and the relationships between generalist and specialist preparation for the discipline. I loved the opportunity for intellectual debate afforded by graduate education in nursing, and longed for more. While I took a 5-year hiatus from my own academic studies in order to practice as a public health and community mental health nurse, I maintained academic ties to the University. I participated as a clinical faculty member supervising students in the graduate program in psychiatric mental health nursing, took some courses as a part-time student, and always "hung around" with nurses from the University. I found colleagues among the nurses who were on the faculty. I knew then that I needed to pursue doctoral education in nursing. Before doing so, I explored the programs around the country. I chose to pursue the PhD in nursing at New York University as I believed that it was the most academically challenging program at the time. It was everything I expected it to be—academic discourse, cutting edge science and research, interesting and challenging academic role models, and, importantly for me, intellectually challenging on a personal level. I learned the academic role as scholar and teaching through observing others and having the opportunity to practice as a junior faculty member.

Mentors

I have had many mentors throughout my academic career. One of my first mentors continues as a mentor today. Grayce Sills was on the faculty at Ohio State University School of Nursing when I was a master's prepared community mental health nurse practicing in Columbus Ohio. She took me under her wing and provided guidance to me in both my academic and professional nursing development. Grayce took me to my first professional association meeting and I have been a professional association "junkie" ever since. She introduced me to the politics of professional nursing, as she had been guided by Hildegard Peplau, one of the masters of professional organization politics. When it came time to choose a doctoral program in nursing, it was Grayce who steered me to NYU and Martha Rogers, suggesting that I would resonate with the advanced and radical thought emanating from NYU. I was never sorry that I followed that advice.

My second set of mentors were found at NYU; both Martha Rogers and Florence Downs guided me in different ways and different directions. Martha stretched my conceptual and professional thinking, pushing the boundaries of the discipline intellectually and practically. I was always amazed at the integrity that she displayed in all that she did. Florence served as my research adviser and introduced me to the rigors of research so important in scientific nursing both then and now.

My third set of professional mentors were introduced to me in my first academic position following my doctoral degree. I assumed a position of leadership in theory and research in academic nursing and sought out the mentorship of Harriet Werley, who at that time, in my mind, was the founder of nursing research in the U.S. As a new faculty member I introduced myself to Harriet and told her that I wanted to know everything that she knew about nursing research. She took me under her wing as a coeditor in the design and launch of the *Annual Review of Nursing Research* series (now in its 22nd volume), with the understanding that I would assume leadership for the series within a 5-year period. Unlike my other mentors, Harriet's training had been in the discipline of psychology, which had a rich history of academic development in research, teaching, and clinical practice. This mentorship provided grounding for me in the inclusion of all of these components.

ENHANCED DEVELOPMENT OF MY TEACHING AND LEADERSHIP SKILLS

Timing is everything, and the timing of my introduction to academic nursing at the doctoral level was critical to my own development as a teacher. Immediately after completing my PhD in nursing I accepted a faculty position in a school of nursing that had just developed a doctoral program in nursing. I was asked to teach the first course, the introduction to nursing theory and research. In the first course, I had 5 doctoral students and 5 faculty members as students. One of the faculty members was a full professor in the school of nursing, and I learned very early that I had expertise that was different and important to the discipline of nursing. I learned to believe in my own expertise. Because I was the only faculty member with a doctoral degree in nursing, I learned quickly to clarify the need for development of graduate education (particularly doctoral education) within the discipline to develop our science, rather than to borrow all of our knowledge from other disciplines. My teaching was refined because it was challenged; this undoubtedly influenced my evolution as a teacher.

I have always felt a high level of comfort as a teacher. In fact, I am more comfortable each year. The more experience I have as a teacher, the better I am as a teacher. This degree of comfort is not always translated into formal presentations. I still experience a degree of discomfort whenever doing a formal presentation. I am not sure why this is the case.

CHALLENGES AND REWARDS

One of my challenges as a teacher is no doubt the challenge of many of my colleagues. That is, the difficulty inherent in balancing all that we have to do as leaders in academic nursing: teaching, writing, researching, and advising students at all levels. Every day requires a juggling of priorities, in which the decision that is made often is based on the greatest good for the greatest number of persons. Yet, on a day-to-day level, sometimes these decisions are not as clear-cut as they appear. Another challenge is the realization that there is no "down time" as an academic leader . . . years later will quote your communication to them. I learned early in my academic career that there is no such thing as casual conversation.

One of the most rewarding aspects of teaching is to see the success of one's students. I have had hundreds of successful students over the course of my many years of teaching. Many of these students are in key positions of leadership in nursing throughout the world. I chose nursing education as an area of focus because I believed that the ripple effect was so important. I can influence the health of so many more people by influencing the high level education of many nurses. Teaching future teachers of nurses and preparing future leaders in nursing is very rewarding to me.

One of my concerns over my years as a teacher has been the parochial views within the ranks of nurses themselves. We have the potential to determine our own destiny, but often do not exercise the potential. The lack of intellectual discourse, challenges to the system, and acceptance of the status quo are frustrating to me. I wish nurse faculty members were more likely to be risk takers, asking questions that are visionary and future oriented rather than continuing the present state of learning.

CONTINUING GROWTH FOR SELF AND OTHERS

I try to learn something new every day, by reading, by listening to experts from outside and inside of nursing and health care. I have always believed that the more exposure to information the better. I am an avid consumer of all that is available on the Internet. I try to learn from information that is available in a range of sources. The amount of health care information available to all of us is overwhelming; it is difficult to discern what information is most critical. But the more you know the easier it is to discern the value of information.

I also try to network with as many people as possible, on the local, national, and global level. I keep a wide range of contacts, particularly within nursing circles. I spend a lot of time communicating with other nurses and other health care professionals who have expertise that I do not have.

My advice to new teachers is to continue to learn by trying new methods and techniques of teaching, and do not be afraid to challenge the system. Make certain that you are an avid learner and that you surround yourself with those who can stretch your own development.

CHAPTER 24

Mary Jane Smith

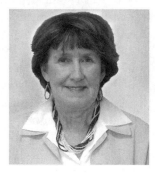

Reflecting on one's personal story of teaching provides an opportunity to consider professional turning points, encourage openness to change, and enable development of one's teaching. Every teacher has a story that describes the way in which their teaching has developed over the years. Story is a way of creating meaning about connections between significant events, as past and future are linked in the present. The construction of a story is a natural human process that enables the understanding of experiences (Smith & Liehr, 2003). When events are remembered and organized in the unfolding story of teaching there is a telling of what was and can be, all in the context of the present moment of the story. This chapter presents the author's story of teaching 30 years of nursing science to master's and doctoral students, and offers examples of significant story-moments in a life of teaching. Through reflection on the experience of teaching core nursing science courses significant story-moments were identified. These story-moments are shifts that seemed to shape and transform teaching. In the process of reflecting on teaching, insights were discerned as the experience of teaching was uncovered. McAdams (1993) believes that human identity is based on "the idea that each of us comes to know who he or she is by creating a story of self" (p. 11).

In reflecting on this personal story, four shifts in the evolution of my experience of teaching surfaced. These shifts are: a) wanting to teach yet not being sure; b) moving along by taking it on; c) letting go and trusting the process; and d) still figuring it out and creating anew. The story that follows is structured by these shifts, which highlight the story-moments as turning points in the developing story of teaching.

WANTING TO TEACH YET NOT BEING SURE

This phase in my life of teaching included these story-moments: letting others do it, attending to a beam of light, and deciding to radiate a lesson. The story begins as I embarked with a new PhD into teaching master's students in a graduate nursing science course. There was a yearning to get the knowledge across and at the same time, a sense of not being sure. Letting others do it was safe, sure, and grounded in the way I was taught in my master's program. At that time, the nursing courses were a series of guest lecturers and student presentations. The teacher of the course coordinated the coming in and the going out of various persons who talked primarily about areas in which they held specialized knowledge. Although the teacher of the course encouraged questions and clarified areas that were not clear, the teacher sat rather passively on the sidelines letting others do the teaching. Certainly one's history and experience as a learner has a deep and powerful impact on the way one teaches. These formative experiences pattern teaching practices. And so, when I began teaching, the class sessions were scheduled with guest lectures, films, and student presentations. At a tacit level, I knew there was something not right about this way of doing things.

During this time, which was in the first 1 or 2 years, I was walking through the hall at the University at a time when classes were going on. The door to a classroom was open, and I heard a faculty lecturing with conviction, as though the point being made was valued and significant. This was a moment of awakening. I said to myself, "A teacher should teach." At that moment—and although it happened long ago I recall it vividly today—I decided to take charge of and responsibility for the courses I was teaching.

I came to grips with the idea of a lesson and began thinking about the course as a series of lessons aimed at meeting the objectives. There was something important to be learned, and conceptualizing what was important up front as it was developed and integrated with previous lessons became my goal. I put together the lesson in detail on 5x8 cards and then presented the lesson to the class. By this I mean, I lectured. The students seemed to be paying attention as they busily took notes. During this phase, there was a progression from sitting on the periphery, more or less as a spectator letting others teach various aspects of the course, to making a decision about teaching with responsibility and conviction.

MOVING ALONG BY TAKING IT ON

This phase of teaching included these story-moments: grasping the lesson of the lesson and actualizing a glimpse of meaning through critical dialogue. The lesson of the lesson came when I read the students' papers and found that many did not get the lesson. Their writing about the major concepts articulated in the lesson lacked breadth, depth, and creativity. The lessons were not taking. I assumed that the students were learning what was being told to them in the lecture and was disappointed with evidence to the contrary. There was a gap in what the teacher assumed was taught and what the students were learning. Brookfield (1995) describes teaching innocently as "assuming that the meanings and significance we place on our actions are the ones that students take from them" (p. 2). Although I had a clear grasp of the meaning to be transmitted in the lesson and the meaning was articulated in a logical way, the lesson did not take. I recall discussing this dilemma with colleagues. One of them sent me a cartoon titled, "How to teach a cow a damned good lesson." It was a depiction of a cow being hit by a two-by-four with the tag line, "First you have to get her attention." It was my belief that I had the students' attention, but I needed to understand why the lesson wasn't taking.

When talking to students about their papers, I could see that they were grappling with creating meaning about the major ideas of the course, and that they were trying to figure things out. There was a yearning to understand and when the yearning was mobilized through discussion, learning was enhanced. It was during this time that I began to feel grounded in what I was doing and how I was thinking about that which I was teaching. Through making clear to students where I was coming from, it began to dawn on me that dialogue between teacher and student, student and student, and student and self were essential to mobilizing a yearning to learn and understand. It was at this time that I attended a seminar given by Richard Paul who believes that critical thinking entails critical questioning. He made the point that although critical thinking is expected, it must be developed and requires effort on the part of the teacher to engage the student in thinking critically. This represented a shift from giving the lesson to critically thinking about the lesson. Paul (1993) describes Socratic questioning as essential to engaging the students in critical thinking. I began thinking about the lesson as a series of questions that would guide the students in thinking through the lesson. These questions took the form of clarifying, raising basic issues, probing, and guiding students through their viewpoints, perspectives, and reasoning as they arrived at a stand in relation to the question. The focal questions for each lesson were outlined on the course syllabus and students were encouraged to read and come to class prepared to discuss the questions with the teacher and with each other. This way of teaching not only took time and energy in preparation, but also a sensitivity in knowing when to push further and when to loosen a bit. This way of engaging dialogue is not so much about finding a right answer and certainly not about one or two word responses, but rather about staying with the question and with the student in order to uncover a deeper understanding of the topic under study. It is essential that the teacher be knowledgeable about the disciplinary perspective that is at the heart of the lesson and be gentle with the students in the critical questioning process. Students often find the questioning disconcerting at the beginning. However, as time goes on, they learn that it is through the questioning that they come to know and understand. A typical student response to the questioning process is, "Calling on students to answer is a good way to get everyone involved. Although I can't say I like being called on (even though it is getting better), the questions make me think a little harder about the subject matter. Knowing I might need to discuss a question in class, I prepare differently." When students are thinking harder, they are more likely to grasp the lesson of the lesson and engage in critical dialogue. In taking on teaching, there was a commitment to build value in each lesson by working steadily, with openness, persistence, and a gentle determination.

LETTING GO AND TRUSTING THE PROCESS

This phase of teaching includes these story-moments: engaging mutual inquiry and enlightenment, and recognizing the unfinished nature of the lesson. In this phase, I was challenged to be truly present in the here and now with students by striving to see and hear their point of view and helping them to expand their view in greater breadth and depth. Kolb (1984) believes that individuals form abstract concepts and generalizations by reflecting on their experience. Changing the way students understand and know nursing comes as they integrate what they are learning with what they already know. Integration is accomplished by engaging students in the critical reflective process of linking their experience with the formation of abstract concepts. I began requiring that students respond to the following statements based on Brookfield's (1995) critical incident format. The questions students respond to in writing are: 1) Describe the time that you were most engaged in class today, 2) Describe the time that you were most distanced in class today, 3) Describe the action that anyone took that was most help-ful to you in class today, 4) Describe the action that anyone took that was most confusing to you today, and 5) What about class surprised you the most today? The students reflect on the class and describe in detail their re-sponses to the questions. For example, in describing when they were most engaged, they are encouraged to elaborate by clarifying and putting in their words what was engaging, and by probing their engagement in light of as-sumptions and viewpoints that they hold. The students e-mail their re-sponse 2 to 3 days after class. The teacher then reads the reflections for common themes and takes time at the beginning of the next class session to discuss the themes with the students. This provides an opportunity for students to hear the reflection of others. Student responses at the end of the course indicate that the reflections have contributed to their integration of the course concepts and to an internalization of the process of critical re-flection. Some written responses that demonstrate an integration of the process of critical thinking and reflection are as follows:

I have been encouraged to think critically; at first I didn't recognize the teaching for what it was. I had to think and stay focused during class. Preparation is key. No easy answers were given to me as I was guided and encouraged to think through the process.

I gained a lot of insight. The reflections were really helpful in my abil-ity to process what I had learned in class.

This course was challenging and the reflections helped me to make sense of the concepts. I will continue to work on applying these concepts in my practice.

In this phase, the challenge of engaging mutual inquiry leads to reflec-tion about what is, what can be, and other questions. Mutual inquiry max-imizes a depth of knowledge and understanding for students and teacher.

STILL FIGURING IT OUT AND CREATING ANEW

In this, the now phase of my life as a teacher, I continue to prepare the teaching/learning session by thinking through the logic of the structure of the session, changing it, and trying to improve the substance, clarity, and integration of the last session. Even though I have been teaching for a long time, there is still the unsettled anticipation of the teaching/learning ses-sion. One never has it down-pat; there is always the yearning to make the teaching/learning session different and to really connect with the students. I think about how I can query the various dimensions of a concept with the students by asking questions about assumptions, meaning, and frame of reference. In addition, I let the students know I expect them to come prepared to discuss, question, and be questioned. Questioning in a nonthreatening manner with the intent to explore the area is always with me in the teaching/learning situation. My intention is not about rightness or wrongness but rather about exploration and discussion. It is this process of discovery that leads to the student's integration of concepts and principles, a deepened understanding, and self-illumination that can be taken on to application. I am always working toward guiding the student in understanding abstract concepts that can be applied in nursing practice.

Another aspect of where I am now is becoming more aware of my presence with students that is beyond instructing and questioning. I am aware that when I come to the teaching/learning situation fully prepared and the students too have read and come prepared, we enter what Bache (2000) refers to as the "Dance of Content and Resonance" (p. 4). In this dance, time passes quickly as ideas and insights come to the group that really spark learning for student and teacher. In the dance, there is an intellectual exchange that goes beyond, to the experience of delight and genuine learning. The dance does not happen in every teaching/learning session and when it does, it is wonderful. Another part of the dance is an other-regarding approach as a way of being teacher that brings a spirit of thoughtfulness and consideration to the students' concerns, problems, and questions in the teaching/learning situation. This approach goes beyond politeness and civility to a genuine presence that seeks first to understand where the student is coming from, to stay with and true to where they are, to move with them to some resolution, and to validate what is understood. I call this an other-regarding approach because as teacher, one chooses deliberately to stay with the student in moving on, through, and beyond as learning and understanding transpires. Taking on an other- regarding approach may not be for everyone; it is how I continue to explore my way of becoming truly myself and finding my own voice as teacher with students.

CONCLUSION

This story came from reflection on turning points in my experience as a teacher of graduate students. The recollective process enabled me to think about those moments in my life as a teacher that mobilized change. It is not so much a story about the what of teaching, although that is important and is the backdrop of the story, but rather a story about engaging the process of teaching. The story is about being present with students through discussion and writing in a way that enables them to think, read, and write critically.

Writing this story has enabled me to claim what I have lived as a teacher and to integrate more fully those insights learned along the way into my present teaching. There is always more to the story and one can never tell the whole story. It is the one recollected. Every teacher is unique and has an original story to recollect and tell. Telling stories is a creative and energizing way to make teaching accessible to ourselves and to others. This story of teaching is shared in the spirit expressed by Nouwen (1997), "We have to trust that our stories deserve to be told. We may discover that the better we tell our stories the better we will want to live them" (p. 5). Telling and listening to stories offer a powerful resource for developing the art of teaching. Stories about teaching are works in progress, worth telling, and worth hearing. These stories are opportunities for sharing attributes about teaching that can make a difference in the lives of students and in the lives of teachers.

REFERENCES

Bache, C. M. (2000). What is transformational learning? *Institute of Noetic Sciences Newsletter,* 2–6.

Brookfield, S. D. (1995). *Becoming a critically reflective teacher.* San Francisco: Jossey-Bass.

Kolb, D. A. (1984). *Experiential learning: Experience as the source of learning and development.* Englewood Cliffs: Prentice-Hall.

McAdams, D. P. (1993). *The stories we live by.* New York: William Morrow.

Nouwen, H. J. (1997). *Bread for the journey.* San Francisco: Harper-Collins.

Paul, R. (1993). *Critical thinking: How to prepare students for a rapidly changing world.* Santa Rosa: Foundation for Critical Thinking.

Smith, M. J., & Liehr, P. (2003). The theory of attentively embracing story. In M. J. Smith & P. L. Liehr (Eds.), *Middle range theory in nursing* (pp. 167–187). New York: Springer Publishing.

CHAPTER 25

Tips and Techniques for Teachers

An important component of our work in preparing this book was to conduct a survey of teachers and students. We knew that there would be richness in the voices of those who were presently engaged in the teaching/learning process. As a course is developed over time, teachers identify and test strategies to make the course better. These strategies then become tried and true tips and techniques that, when made available to others, can be a valuable resource. Our contact with students and teachers was not designed as a research project, but rather as an effort to go into the field and gather the teaching/learning activities of the participants. We believe that the teaching/learning tips and techniques offered by faculty and students will be instructive to others, including new and experienced teachers.

New teachers may wish to first peruse the list and choose several that they may not have thought about but seem to be good ideas that fit the course. Second, they may include the activity throughout the design of the course and accompanying learning activities, and lastly they may use the content to evaluate the effectiveness of the incorporated activity. For example, if a teacher is teaching a distance education course, he or she might choose to focus on integrating activities that foster student interaction with faculty and peers. In thinking through the question about how to foster interaction with students who may be located across the United States and abroad, the teacher might include having the students send a picture, and ask them to write a personal biography at the beginning of the course. With students' permission, both of these activities could also be shared with the other students in the course. In the middle of the course, the students could be asked to share with the teacher and other students a story about their skills and talents, including what they are really good at doing and an area in which they could help one of their classmates. In addition, students could be placed in groups of four to six and, as a group, asked to critique the strengths and shortcomings of an article. Part of this activity is for each student to e-mail the teacher an evaluation of the extent to which each member of the group participated in creating the critique.

Another possibility for use of the listing of tips and techniques is for a teacher to ask "what if" questions in relation to each of the entries on the list. What if I implemented this activity in my course? What specific learning approaches could I incorporate into the course? Trying new techniques and then having the students in their classes evaluate the effectiveness may offer an opportunity to make a small change in the course, that could lead to enhanced student learning along with greater faculty and student satisfaction with the course.

Experienced teachers are always looking for different ways of teaching their classes. They can benefit from the list supplied by others. One example from the list that an experienced teacher may wish to put in place is the one on engaging students in active learning. Even though the experienced teacher uses active learning, ways to enhance this vital aspect of the students' experience is always a goal. In a distance course, this approach uses time with students in synchronous sessions such as chat rooms or in a real time web-cast to discuss what has been assigned as a reading or archived lecture. Posing questions that are focused on the course content and that generate thinking engages the student to become actively involved in his or her learning. When the teacher demonstrates a disciplined critical thought process in gently guiding the students in and through the various responses to the question, active learning is enhanced.

It is our expectation that the list will generate dialogue among faculty colleagues teaching similar courses. For example, faculty teaching research courses at all levels of the curriculum could go through the list and discuss how they incorporate the tips and techniques in their different research courses. This dialogue would not only spawn new and different approaches for each level of the course and may also differentiate the tips and techniques at each level of the course.

Graduate students in nursing education may benefit the most from the lists of tips and techniques. They have an extended opportunity to debate the pros and cons of the various suggestions, to understand them in relation to educational theory, and to consider the categorical structures that would help others to understand the lists. For example, Chickering and Gamson (1991) have delineated 7 principles for good practice for undergraduate teaching. These principles have been studied in a number of undergraduate venues and could provide a method of systematically studying the tips and techniques that were generated by our limited survey. Although the principles have not been studied in graduate education or with selected forms of education such as distance or intensive courses, it could be the project of graduate students to discern how the list of tips and techniques in these selected areas apply to the Chickering and Gamson (1991) principles. These 7 principles of good teaching are as follows:

1. Good practice encourages student-faculty contact.
2. Good practice encourages cooperation among students and colleagues.
3. Good practice encourages active learning.
4. Good practice gives prompt feedback.
5. Good practice emphasizes time on task.
6. Good practice communicates high expectations.
7. Good practice respects diverse talents and ways of learning and teaching. (Chickering & Gamson, 1991)

In our surveys, we obtained comments from both faculty and students in the following types of courses: intensive graduate level nursing courses, clinical nursing courses (both undergraduate and graduate), distance nursing courses (both undergraduate and graduate), and nursing research courses (both undergraduate and graduate). In addition, we asked students what meaningful advice teachers had given to them. Our first approach was to try to categorize and organize the various tips and techniques. In fact, we pursued several versions of categories. In the final analysis we decided to present the data, in the words of the students and the faculty, so that the reader might be exposed to the richness of these data. Each of the sections below is preceded by a short introduction.

COMMENTS FROM FACULTY AND STUDENTS IN INTENSIVE COURSES

Intensive courses are those offered in a condensed or executive format. For example, classes might be held for 6 days in a row, or for 3 days each weekend for two weekends in a row. Often the didactic component of the course is offered in this condensed time frame and the students have follow-up time to complete the course assignments. Faculty were asked to provide tips and techniques for intensive courses, and to indicate what does not work in intensive courses. Students were asked what teachers do to help them learn and what teachers do that does not help them learn.

TABLE 25.1 Intensive Course: Faculty Teaching Tips and Techniques

Tips and Techniques to Help Students Learn

- Allow library time for student preparation of presentations
- Attend to compressed format of an intensive course
- Balance an informal and formal teaching style
- Balance heavy and light content
- Be flexible and fair to all students
- Be positive
- Be realistic about amount of content given to students
- Build on students' life and professional experiences
- Communicate clear expectations that remain in place throughout the course
- Communicate frequently
- Develop a peer feedback system to get constructive feedback from students
- Discuss students' questions completely
- Display a sense of humor
- Do a summary evaluation of class session at end of each day
- Engage students in learning through projects
- Get to know the students
- Interject human interest stories
- Involve physical activity in teaching modalities
- Let student discussion evolve
- Prepare for students who register at the last minute
- Prepare for the class
- Promote an environment of partnership between students and faculty
- Provide a "roadmap" to identify the direction of the course
- Provide multiple short breaks
- Provide the syllabus 4–6 weeks ahead of time
- Recognize student energy lags
- Select self-motivated adult learners for the course

(continued)

TABLE 25.1 Intensive Course: Faculty Teaching Tips and Techniques (*Continued*)

- Structure plans for negotiating an incomplete course grade
- Take brain breaks frequently
- Take care of yourself
- Understand the intensive teaching modality
- Use a variety of classroom approaches, including debates and class presentations
- Use a variety of teaching techniques
- Use active learning strategies
- Use an occasional guest speaker
- Use available course management systems
- Use blackboard, e-mail, and phone as means of communication
- Use multiple teaching strategies
- Use the time-honored tradition of food wisely
- Websites are available to all students

Intensive Faculty Perspectives of What Does Not Work

- Allowing too much time before assignments are due
- Attempt to use same format and assignments as regular semester course
- Failure to provide syllabus ahead of time
- Lack of preparation
- Not enough structure
- Not varying the teaching methods
- Too rigid
- Class size not large enough

TABLE 25.2 Intensive Course: Students' Perspectives

Students' Perspectives of What Teachers Do to Help Them Learn

- Act as role model for professional life/development
- Be available to answer questions outside of the classroom
- Demonstrate knowledge of the course material
- Discuss how to write for publication
- Display qualities of a master teacher
- Focus on learning, not assignments
- Give a template for identifying learning needs
- Have a positive attitude
- Have a sense of humor

(continued)

TABLE 25.2 Intensive Course: Students' Perspectives (*Continued*)

- Help students in the process of discovery
- Offer a variety of teaching methods
- Provide a comfortable and conducive learning environment
- Provide a sense of the whole—the big picture
- Provide a collegial atmosphere
- Provide encouragement
- Provide flexibility in learning activities
- Provide positive feedback and reinforcement
- Provide skillful guidance
- Provide small group discussions
- Serve as a guide for learning
- Share ideas and information
- Show advanced knowledge and enthusiasm
- Show genuine interest in the students and subject matter
- Show importance of engaging students
- Summarize main ideas
- Teach the process of scholarly writing
- Tell stories
- Use clinical examples, case studies, and visual aids
- Use multiple teaching modalities

Students' Perspectives of What Teachers Do That Does Not Help Them Learn

- Displaying the fact that they are burned out
- Failing to be engaged in the course
- Failing to integrate guest speaker content into the course
- Failing to provide course materials in a timely manner
- Imparting the feeling that this is just his/her job
- Lack of preparation
- Not able to move beyond their own work
- Providing unclear directions for assignments
- Using too many guest speakers

COMMENTS FROM FACULTY AND STUDENTS IN CLINICAL COURSES

Clinical courses consisted of courses in which there was a clinical component in addition to the didactic component. Both undergraduate and graduate faculty and students were surveyed. Faculty were asked to provide tips and techniques for clinical courses, and also to indicate what does not work in clinical courses. Students were asked what teachers do to help them learn and what teachers do that does not help them learn.

TABLE 25.3 Clinical Course: Faculty Teaching Tips and Techniques

Tips and Techniques to Help Students Learn

- Address student fears and earn trust and respect
- Be patient and offer guidance to enhance student learning
- Case presentation
- Case studies
- Case studies with simulated patients
- Challenge but do not overwhelm students with a clinical assignment
- Clinical conferences
- Communicate the plan for each class, including break times
- Communicate via e-mail to post announcements and changes in the schedule
- Competency-based education tools
- Convey a nonthreatening demeanor
- Create a nurturing environment
- Create learning experiences where students are not bogged down by staff demands
- Demonstration lectures
- Demonstrations
- Discuss case scenarios
- Do not give all the lecture notes to students ahead of time, so that they are encouraged to pay attention
- Evaluate strengths and weakness of each student daily
- Examples from clinical practice
- Faculty engagement with students
- Foster self-esteem
- Get to know students before taking them to the clinical area
- Give a practice math test so students know what to expect
- Give clear guidelines and expectations
- Give constructive feedback with specificity on how to improve
- Grade contracting
- Group learning
- Guide independent practice of procedures before clinical application
- Guide students to assess and document from a holistic perspective

(continued)

TABLE 25.3 Clinical Course: Faculty Teaching Tips and Techniques (*Continued*)

- Guide students to identify their own learning needs and set goals for their clinical day
- Guide students to not prejudge patients
- Help students analyze their thinking underlying an error that they have made
- Help students learn to think for themselves by being accountable as caregivers
- Implement roundtable discussion after each clinical course, where students share salient experiences
- Include stories from the teacher's practice that illustrate important points
- Include student exercises as part of the class
- Include visuals in presentations
- Involve students in learning
- Lecture
- Maintain good relationships with clinical staff so that the environment is supportive of learning
- Morning rounds to each assigned client
- Ongoing student evaluation with a great deal of feedback, both positive and developmental
- Participate as an expert in the practice area where students are learning
- Point out subtle differences in practice
- Power Point presentations with handouts of the slides as study guides
- Practice so that the teacher walks the walk as well as talks the talk
- Practice what is preached
- Preceptorships in clinical setting
- Proofread and edit notes with the student before they are written on the chart
- Provide a nurturing environment
- Provide clear objectives
- Provide handouts for students
- Provide a highly structured environment
- Provide opportunities for students to learn from each other as well as from the teacher
- Provide opportunities for students to observe the teacher in practice
- Provide repeated exposure to important content
- Provide students with opportunities to explore many ways of intervening
- References, including Web resources
- Reinforcement of learning
- Repeat very important points several times through out the lecture
- Respect each student

(continued)

TABLE 25.3 Clinical Course: Faculty Teaching Tips and Techniques (*Continued*)

- Role model interactions with students and patients
- Role-play
- Schedule a test review session after each test so students can evaluate their own learning
- Sequence learning tasks
- Show enthusiasm for teaching
- Spend time in pre-conference reviewing each student's care plan for the day
- Stay available to the student
- Stay current in practice
- Student presentations
- Support student self-evaluation on a weekly basis
- Take time to help students with a procedure by guiding them through it
- Team building activities
- Tell stories
- Use a scavenger hunt to orient students to the new hospital unit
- Use as many pictures as possible in Power Point slides
- Use contracting for student learning
- Use experts
- Use humor when possible
- Use journaling
- Use multiple teaching modalities
- Use pictures from the Web
- Use simulations
- Use Socratic method to assist students to develop problem solving skills
- Use the Internet
- When many students fail to perform as the teacher expects, review in detail information they have been given
- Work with students in order to provide a richer clinical experience

Clinical Faculty Perspectives of What Does Not Work

- A clinical environment that promotes fear
- All lecture, all of the time
- Clinical objectives that are not clearly written
- Enhancing one's power by being overly aggressive with students
- Evaluating students before they have time to learn
- Group projects where some do more of their share of work and others do less

(*continued*)

TABLE 25.3 Clinical Course: Faculty Teaching Tips and Techniques (*Continued*)

- Increasing student anxiety by talking down to students and being overly critical
- Instructor who is not clinically competent
- Instructor who lets the students go at their own pace
- Lack of patience in guiding students
- Long class days
- Long videotaped lectures
- Prejudging a student by appearance or rumors from other faculty
- Providing expectations that are not clear
- Surprises on clinical evaluation because students have been mislead by positive faculty remarks
- Class size too large
- Videos longer than 5–10 minutes

TABLE 25.4 Clinical Course: Students' Perspectives

Students' Perspectives of What Teachers Do to Help Them Learn

- Answer questions in detail
- Apply text material to real life situations through examples
- Are clear about expectations
- Are organized and prepared for learning experience
- Are patient and let the student work through problems without telling the answers
- Ask questions to focus the group on discussion
- Ask the question, "Why?"
- Build trust in the teacher-student relationship
- Discuss clinical situations, including what to do and why the steps are important
- Discuss student strengths and weaknesses individually
- Display an open personality
- Encourage involvement and interaction
- Encourage students by telling them that they are doing a good job
- Engage in one-to-one discussion
- Expect the most from students
- Explain equipment in detail
- Facilitate learning
- Focus on student success
- Functions as a role model that shows students how to practice
- Give immediate feedback

(continued)

TABLE 25.4 Clinical Course: Students' Perspectives *(Continued)*

- Go into the patient's room with the student for the first few times
- Have a knowledge base and expertise
- Have students exchange experiences at the end of each clinical day
- Help students focus on the patient from a holistic perspective
- Help students to go beyond the traditional textbook
- Incorporate different learning methods
- Offer constructive criticism
- Patiently talk the student through performance of a procedure
- Provide copies of notes and stick to the syllabus
- Provide framework for learning and expectations
- Provide hands-on experiences
- Provide nursing knowledge and reinforce theory with an emphasis on critical thinking
- Provide office hours
- Provide study guides to show important information
- Relate clinical stories and connect the story to what is being studied
- Relieve stress through humor, caring, and compassion
- Remain calm
- Review procedures with students before entering the patient's room
- Start discussions that make you think
- Stay focused on topic content
- Tell stories about real patients
- Use case studies incorporating theory and critical thinking to arrive at a solution
- Use variety of resources
- Use visual tools
- Willing to work one-on-one with students

Students' Perspectives of What Teachers Do That Does Not Help Them Learn

- Adding to the students' nervousness
- Not being approachable
- Assuming everyone knows the terminology
- Assuming students already know the content
- Assume students have acquired information in past courses
- Being unprepared
- Breathing down students back by staring at them
- Correcting students by yelling at them in front of the patient and family

(continued)

TABLE 25.4 Clinical Course: Students' Perspectives (*Continued*)

- Demeaning students
- Drawing lectures from limited resources
- Expecting students to read the teacher's mind
- Expecting the student to answer a question quickly
- Failing to explain concepts related to the slides
- Failing to use current technology
- Not having patience with students
- Injecting negativity into the learning experience
- Involving students in group work when the information needed to do the work is not provided
- Lecturing all of the time
- Making students buy five textbooks and only use one of them
- Omitting practical information in clinical course lectures
- Not providing enough lecture time on assigned readings
- Not providing more days and longer hours for clinical practice
- Reading from lecture notes
- Reading from Power Point slides
- Requiring study guides for each of the areas covered in the course
- Requiring too much reading
- Straying from topic
- Telling student to "figure it out"
- Throwing students into unexpected situations
- Use of negative talk

COMMENTS FROM FACULTY AND STUDENTS IN DISTANCE EDUCATION COURSES

Distance education courses were those in which the course was offered with a physical distance between faculty and students, through interactive Web-based learning or through the use of other technology. Faculty were asked to provide tips and techniques for distance education courses, and also to indicate what does not work in distance education courses. Students were asked what teachers do to help them learn and what teachers do that does not help them learn.

TABLE 25.5 Distance Course: Faculty Teaching Tips and Techniques

Tips and Techniques to Help Students Learn

- Anticipate problems with the technology
- Avoid communicating unnecessary information and communicate often
- Be available
- Call on students who do not respond in the chat room
- Check all websites to which you refer students
- Create diverse course activities
- Demonstrate mutual respect for other faculty team members
- Demonstrate proficiency with information technology
- Develop teaching skills
- Engage the students in active learning
- Get to know the students
- Give detailed and specific instructions
- Identify a portion of class grade for participation
- Integrate activities that foster student interaction with faculty and peers
- Limit number of students in a chat room
- Link to other on-line information
- Offer synchronous group work assignments
- Participate as teacher and producer of the course
- Plan content from back to front
- Post the structural components of the course
- Post weekly course notes
- Promote student peer support
- Provide active learning activities
- Provide clear on-line instructions for each assignment
- Provide framework for student lifelong learning
- Provide group work on-line
- Provide rapid response to questions
- Provide step-by-step plan for student success
- Put faculty and student addresses on the webpage
- Require group work and projects
- Require weekly reflections
- Review course content
- Seek peer support and feedback
- Use all of the facilities and resources available

(continued)

TABLE 25.5 Distance Course: Faculty Teaching Tips and Techniques (*Continued*)

- Use case studies and scenerios
- Use exercises to help the students learn on-line technology

Distance Faculty Perspectives of What Does Not Work

- Assigning an excessive amount of work
- Avoiding long explanations of assignments
- Displaying indifference to students
- Failure to attend to student group participation
- Giving busywork to students
- Posting unrelated materials on the course website
- Treating the course as self-study rather than distance education
- Using excessive Power Point slides
- Using passive learning strategies
- Waiting until the last minute to put course materials on-line

TABLE 25.6 Distance Course: Students' Perspectives

Students' Perspectives of What Faculty Do to Help Them Learn

- Be as clear as possible about what is expected
- Discuss various topics on a discussion board so that all can see the discussion
- Encourage open communication
- Encourage student responsibility for assignments
- Give direction for further development
- Give feedback on work that has been completed
- Touch base with students frequently
- Keep students involved in learning by asking poll questions
- Make course announcements available to everyone
- Provide timely responses to questions
- Provide detailed written responses to assignments
- Provide for interaction with all members of the class
- Provide on-line opportunities for student contact outside of class
- Provide students with a way to reach each other in the class
- Recognize busy schedules of students
- Repeat questions before giving the answer
- Space out assignments over the term

(continued)

TABLE 25.6 Distance Course: Students' Perspectives (*Continued*)

Students' Perspectives of What Teachers Do That Does Not Help Them Learn

- Causing anxiety by not answering student questions
- Not communicating with the students regularly
- Not providing feedback
- Not returning assignments or answering questions in a timely manner
- Giving assignments that are difficult to understand
- Giving reading assignments that are overwhelming
- Not being available for immediate personal assistance
- Providing unclear answers to questions
- Putting too much responsibility on the student for learning

COMMENTS FROM FACULTY AND STUDENTS IN RESEARCH COURSES

Research courses were comprised of both undergraduate and graduate courses taught in a traditional classroom format, in which the content was research methods. Faculty were asked to provide tips and techniques for research courses, and also to indicate what does not work in teaching research courses. Students were asked what teachers do to help them learn and what teachers do that does not help them learn.

TABLE 25.7 Research Course: Faculty Teaching Tips and Techniques

Tips and Techniques to Help Students Learn

- Ask questions rather than answering them
- Attend to what students are saying
- Be explicit in instructions at the beginning of the course about expectations and assignments
- Be gently honest about less than excellent work of the students
- Break the research process into smaller steps
- Build a supportive network among the students
- Creatively engage students in learning
- Discuss critiques of articles openly in class
- Distinguish between a clinical problem and a research problem
- Empower students to learn

TABLE 25.7 Research Course: Faculty Teaching Tips and Techniques (*Continued*)

- Encourage attendance at local research conferences
- Encourage attendance at all research conferences
- Encourage students to present at the school research day
- Have students bring an article for discussion that uses the concepts they are interested in exploring
- Have students develop a matrix to delineate the key concepts in a research study
- Help students not be overwhelmed with lots of assignments
- Include how to develop a poster
- Introduce students to doctoral level faculty and their programs of research
- Let students know research is a journey
- Pay attention to critical evaluation in writing
- Present the real with the ideal
- Provide advice about career planning for graduate schools
- Provide for student presentations
- Provide opportunities for students to learn without fear of making mistakes
- Provide opportunities for students to participate in small research projects with faculty guidance
- Share challenges and rewards of research
- Share personal stories about research
- Stress the importance of research for the profession
- Use a research utilization model for addressing course content
- Use discussion techniques that challenge each student
- Use evidence-based practice examples
- Use exercises that accompany course content in textbook
- Use humor
- Use jump ropes, Lego building blocks, or jacks to describe different kinds of research
- Use on-line, open book, open note exams
- Use peer evaluation and peer grading
- Use research critique assignment as the final examination
- Use seminar approach rather than lecture to facilitate interaction

Research Faculty Perspectives of What Does Not Work

- Requiring too many articles for critique
- Requiring too many assignments, so that students think research is labor intensive and boring
- Speaking over the heads of students
- Straight lecture

TABLE 25.8 Research Course: Students' Perspectives

Perspectives of What Teachers Do to Help Them Learn

- Answer questions in detail
- Be approachable
- Be understanding
- Compare and contrast research articles
- Concentrate on important points
- Discuss real life research projects
- Encourage attendance at research conferences
- Encourage questions
- Encourage self-learning
- Encourage students to read professional nursing journals
- Explain information carefully
- Explain research utilization
- Explain the process of research in nursing
- Give handouts to reinforce ideas
- Give take-home exercises
- Help students relate research to clinical applications
- Make class interactive
- Offer consistent enthusiasm
- Offer practice questions, and review questions in class
- Present material in a concise and interesting manner
- Provide all assignments at the beginning of the course
- Provide course textbook and all relevant course materials at the beginning of class
- Provide detailed outline and course syllabus
- Provide great slides
- Provide guidance
- Provide learning activities that are unique
- Provide examples from personal research experience
- Provide review materials prior to exams
- Provide specific examples in class
- Provide time outside the classroom for one-to-one involvement
- Provide visual aids
- Relate research concepts to everyday examples
- Repeat important content
- Review important material

(continued)

TABLE 25.8 Research Course: Students' Perspectives *(Continued)*

- Use active learning in the classroom
- Use class discussions
- Use clinical examples in teaching research
- Use interesting and interactive material
- Use Power Point slides judiciously and make these available to students
- Use small group exercises
- Use worksheets

Students' Perspectives of What Teachers Do That Does Not Help Them Learn

- Assigning a lot of reading without noting what is important in the reading
- Being unapproachable
- Covering material too quickly
- Displaying lack of enthusiasm for the subject
- Not providing connections between key concepts
- Not providing time for questions or discussion
- Expressing dissatisfaction with having to teach the class
- Failure to answer questions
- Failure to explain the information
- Failure to explain theories
- Failure to provide adequate explanations
- Going too fast
- Lack of coordination among professors teaching different sections
- Lack of emphasis on application of research
- Lack of opportunity to participate in research
- Lack of respect for students and their questions
- Lack of specificity about course material
- Lack of visual aids
- Long class periods
- Long reading assignments
- Monotone voice
- Moving too slow
- No variation in the way material is presented
- Not enough emphasis on research implementation in the clinical area
- Not enough interactive assignments
- Not providing opportunities for self-learning
- Providing disorganized and unclear lecture

(continued)

TABLE 25.8 Research Course: Students' Perspectives (*Continued*)

- Providing same material as presented in the book
- Providing too much detail about the research
- Reading from the text, Power Point slides, or other course materials
- Shooting down answers
- Too many students in the class
- Using only lecture format
- Using only Power Point to teach with; no group participation

STUDENTS' COMMENTS ABOUT MEANINGFUL ADVICE GIVEN TO THEM BY TEACHERS

All students were asked to tell us what advice they had received from faculty members. Some advice that the students reported having received fell into a category of nursing practice advice. However, the majority of examples given by students fell into a broader category of "life advice." This latter category provides support for the mentoring that is occurring between nurse faculty and students.

TABLE 25.9 Meaningful Advice Given to Students by Teachers

Meaningful Life Advice

- Apply what you have learned
- Appreciate diversity
- Ask colleagues for help or advice
- Ask questions when you do not understand
- Be enthusiastic
- Be kind and respectful to others
- Be open and receptive to learning every day
- Be patient
- Be patient and compassionate with others
- Be prepared
- Communication is essential
- Consider different perspectives
- Do not swallow elephants or choke on gnats
- Do not take yourself too seriously
- Do the best you can

(continued)

TABLE 25.9 Meaningful Advice Given to Students by Teachers (*Continued*)

- Giving up will do you in
- It's OK not to know the answer
- Keep learning
- Learn from mistakes
- Learn something from every experience
- Love what you do and develop your full potential
- Never assume anything
- Never give up on your dream
- Never underestimate yourself
- Organization is important to not losing your mind
- Pursue higher education
- Reach for the stars
- Remain open-minded
- Slow down
- Strive for excellence
- Take advantage of every aspect of learning possible
- Take as much as you can from your current experience
- Take each day as a new day
- Take things one day at a time
- The journey is as important as the destination
- There is never a dumb question; to be dumb is not to ask the question
- Think critically
- Think with an open mind
- Have faith in yourself and trust your judgment
- Never give up on yourself
- Touch the lives of people.
- Use reasoning, common sense, and critical thinking skills
- When you do not succeed the first time, do not settle for less the second time
- Your response is your responsibility
- Your work is not your worth

Meaningful Nursing Practice Advice

- Apply theory to clinical practice
- Assess and reassess your patients
- Do not expect to be an expert about nursing right away
- Document accurately

(continued)

TABLE 25.9 Meaningful Advice Given to Students by Teachers (*Continued*)

- Each patient is a unique individual having had different life experiences from all others
- Every nurse contributes to health care
- It is important to care
- Listen attentively to the patient and family
- Listen to patients and be an advocate
- Listen to patients and be compassionate
- Never let the rules of systems get in the way of excellent nursing practice
- Nurses make a significant difference in someone's life
- Nursing care is important and influences the lives of patients
- Nursing requires flexibility, skills, and confidence
- Performing skills and genuinely caring for patients are important acts
- Realize differences between ideals being taught and the reality of nursing practice
- Teamwork is essential for good patient care
- The art of caring is being truly present
- The rewards of nursing are outstanding
- Things will not always go your way so go on the best way that you can
- Treat patients how you would treat family members
- You can best help a patient when you listen and hear what is said

REFERENCES

Chickering, A. B., & Gamson, Z. F. (Eds.). (1991). Applying the seven principles for good practice in undergraduate education. In *New directions for teaching and learning*. San Francisco: Jossey-Bass.

Acknowledgment
of Survey Participants

FACULTY

Nancy Alfred
Mary Anthony
Mary Ann Cantrell
Laura Clayton
Rose Ann DiMaria
Cindy Drenning
Gloria Fowler
Kimberly Glenn
Michele Godwin
Patricia Higgins
Monica Kennison
Jean Lange
June Larrabee
Patricia Liehr
Elizabeth Madigan
Diana McCarty
Shirley Misselwitz
Reynold Mosier
Susan Newfield
Barbara Nunley
Cynthia Persily
Elise Pizzi
Diane Seibert
Laurie Theeke
Geri Wood
Sarah Wrenn

STUDENTS

Paul Allen
Jennifer Amandus
Shogher Amyan
Lu Attemc
Brandi Ball
Brenna Ball
James Balman
Linda Beechinor
Aliza Ben-Zacharia
Julie Boyden
Joanne Brunet
Sarah Buckley
Barbara Buerke
Colleen Burke
Terry Canter
Crystal Caudio
Chesed Ceniseroz
Sarah Christman
Alaina Christy
Michaela Connolly
Jimy Cook
Danielle Cunningham
Sara Curley
Michelle deCastro
Camlinh Dinh
Becky DiProsperis

Brianne Donahoe
Carol Dwyer
Julie Ebe
Karen Esnes
Jennifer Fedele
Pamela Fernandez
Donna Fitzgerald
Katie Fowle
Vania Fox
Shirley George
Brandi Goss
Nancy Greathouse
Karen Haught
Dan Hayes
Courtney Hoeksema
David Holloway
Katie Jacoly
Heather Johnson
Roxy Kaboli
Barbara Kennedy
Jessica Kerns
Katherine Kiddle
Kyle Kincaid
Christin Kurz
Victoria Latess
Meagan Leahy
Tasha Lucas
Joseph Marcantel
Sandra Martin
Scott Masloski
Anne-Marie McAlarnen
Leah McElroy
Charlene McMenemy
Carelle Jade Medel
Naomi Medley
Ashley Metzler
Kate Murphy
Chris Niles

Julie O'Brien
Maggie O'Connor
Luzuiminda Palad
Jamie Pavlonnis
Carissa Petroro
Kimberly Phillips
Christina Piper
Cortney Poth
Lindsey Reilly
Mark Riedmann
Marni Robbins
Johnny Rollins
Roshann Samuels
Stephanie Sauers
Angela Schaffer
Christy Sevier
Alaysa Simons
Courtney Sisk
Dwayne Smith II
Monica Smith
Stephanie Snouffer
Schelly Snyder
Neive Sparr
Meredith Stauring
Jennifer Stefanik
Jose Tapia
Kristin Tennant
Ross Tennant
Erin Tucker
Jill Tynell
Lauren Visalli
Colleen Walker
James Weed
Nichole Werger
Sharon Weyer
Elizabeth Williams
Jamie Young

Index

Accessibility, teacher–student relationship, 26
Accountability, 64–65
Administrative functions, 16, 107, 160–161
Administrative structure, 7
Adult learners, 151
Ah-ha moments, 106, 159
Allen, David, 143
Angry students, 76
Assignments, 79, 184
Attention-getting strategies, 23
Audience engagement, 51
Austin, Lois, Dr., 10, 12

Balance, importance of, 73, 115, 158, 174
Barber, Janet., 5
Behavioral change, 32
Benner, Patricia, 144
Bevis, Em, 143
Billings, Diane M.
  advice for new teachers, 8
  awards and recognitions, 3
  challenges faced, 6
  early interest in teaching, 4
  educational background, 3
  embarrassing moments, 7
  evolution as a teacher, 5–6
  feeling comfortable, 6
  fellowships, 3
  least rewarding aspects of teaching, 7
  maintaining excellence, 7–8
  mentoring, 5, 64
  preparation for teaching, 4–5
  professional background, 3
  professional memberships, 3
  rewarding aspects of teaching, 7
Brainstorming, 125
Byron, William J., S. J., 14

Career development, 87, 94–95, 116
Change resistance, dealing with, 145
Change theory, 101
Charisma, 152
Chater, Shirley, 140, 142
Cheating students, 123
Chinn, Peggy, 143
Clinical courses, 188–194
Clinical decision making, 141–142
Clinical judgment, 141, 144
Clinical practice, 4, 81
Clinical specialists, 43–44, 101
Coach, teacher as, 54
Cognitive theory, 144
Commitment, importance of, 17, 34, 87, 148, 158
Community health nursing, 15, 118, 120
Community of scholars, 18
Confidence, development of, 46, 60, 80, 148
Confrontation, 123
Consultation, 169
Continuing education, importance of, 7, 17, 96, 103
Contradictions, 93–94
Coulter, Pearl Parvin, 158
Counseling education, 120
Course evaluation, 167, 179–180
Creativity, importance of, 6, 16
Critical analysis, 16

Critical review, 92
Critical thinking skills, 178–180
Cultural diversity, significance of, 16, 74
Curriculum, generally
    changes, impact of, 6–7, 54, 60, 68
    development, 100, 102, 132, 139, 146
Curriculum Revolution, 143

"Dance of Content and Resonance," 181
Dewey, John, 135–136
Dialogue engagement, 178–179
Diekelmann, Nancy, 58, 143
Diers, Donna, 88
Diploma school teaching, 4, 7, 33, 101
Disgruntled students, 76
Disruptive students, 111, 137
Distance education courses, 154, 194–197
Doctoral programs, 7, 11–12, 20, 22,
        40–41, 54–55
Donley, Rosemary, Sister
    advice for new teachers, 18–19
    challenges faced, 15–16
    early interest in teaching, 10
    educational background, 9
    embarrassing moments, 17
    evolution as a teacher, 12–15
    feeling comfortable, 15
    fellowship, 9, 13, 15
    least rewarding aspects of teaching, 16
    maintaining excellence, 17–18
    mentoring, 14, 114
    preparation for teaching, 10–12
    professional background, 9
    professional memberships, 9
    rewarding aspects of teaching, 16
Downs, Florence S.
    advice for new teachers, 28–29
    challenges faced, 25
    early interest in teaching, 21
    educational background, 20
    embarrassing moments, 27
    evolution as a teacher, 22–24
    as facilitator of learning community,
        26–27
    feeling comfortable, 24–25
    least rewarding aspects of teaching, 27
    maintaining excellence, 28
    mentoring, 20, 22, 28–29, 173
    potential development, 25–26
    preparation for teaching, 21–22
    professional background, 20
    professional memberships, 20
    rewarding aspects of teaching, 27
Drennan, Phyllis, 142
Dreyfus, Bert, 143
Dumas, Rhetaugh, 88

Edmondson, Mark, 86
Educational design, 100
Educational research, 69
Educational theory, 39
Effective teacher, characteristics of, 162
Ellis, Patrick, Brother, 14
Enabler, teacher as, 3, 8
Engagement techniques, 72, 89, 101
Enthusiasm, importance of, 161, 166
Erickson, Helen, 121
Ethical responsibility, 125
Evaluation system, 48
Evidence-based practice, 54
Expectations, 79, 85
Experiential learning, 66

Facilitator, teacher as, 3, 8, 26–27, 54–55
Faculty development, 117
Faculty Research Oriented Groups
        (FROG), 112
Faculty roles, 159
Fahey, George, Dr., 12
Failure, student, 35, 66, 137
Feedback, importance of, 48, 50, 105
Fellowship recipients, see specific
        interviewees
Ferguson, Vernice
    advice for new teachers, 36–37
    challenges faced, 34
    early interest in teaching, 31
    educational background, 30
    embarrassing moments, 34
    evolution as a teacher, 32–33
    feeling comfortable, 33
    fellowships, 30, 33
    leadership, 31
    least rewarding aspects of teaching, 35

maintaining excellence, 35–36
mentoring, 32
preparation for teaching, 31–32
professional background, 30, 32–33
professional memberships, 30
rewarding aspects of teaching, 34–35
Field, Bill, 132
Fitzpatrick Joyce J.
    challenges faced, 174
    continual growth, 175
    early interest in teaching, 171
    educational background, 172
    leadership skills, 173–174
    mentoring, 172–173
    rewarding aspects of teaching, 174
    teaching skills, development of,
        173–174
Fitzpatrick, Louise M.
    advice for new teachers, 46–47
    appointments, 38
    challenges faced, 44
    early interest in teaching, 39
    educational background, 38
    educational theory, 39
    embarrassing moments, 44
    evolution as a teacher, 42–44
    feeling comfortable, 44
    fellowships, 38
    least rewarding aspects of teaching, 45
    maintaining excellence, 46
    mentoring, 41–42
    preparation for teaching, 40–41
    professional background, 38, 42–43
    rewarding aspects of teaching, 44–45
Flexibility, 85
Foley, Gertrude, Sister, 14
Frazier, Frances, 40
Frustration, dealing with, 111

Goal-setting, importance of, 148, 159
Grier, Margaret, 144
Ground rules, 79
Group process, 167
Guest speakers/lecturers, 50

Hamilton, Anitta, 63
Hampton, Isabelle, 40

Harcleroad, Fred, Dr., 158
Hassenplug, Lulu Wolf, 157
Heidegger, Martin, 144
Heideggerian hermeneutics, 58
Henderson, Virginia, 87, 89–91
Hickey, Robert, Dr., 13
Holistic healing, 132
Holzemer, William L.
    advice for new teachers, 53–55
    challenges faced, 51–52
    early interest in teaching, 49
    educational background, 48
    embarrassing moments, 52
    evolution as a teacher, 50–51
    feeling comfortable, 51
    fellowships, 48
    least rewarding aspects of teaching,
        52–53
    maintaining excellence, 53
    mentoring, 49–50, 142
    preparation as a teacher, 49
    professional background, 48
    rewarding aspects of teaching, 52
Hostile students, 111
Humility, 133
Humor, importance of, 23, 137, 168–169
Huntsman, Ann, 142

Imposter phenomenon, 90
Integration/synthesis, 133, 140, 179
Integrity, importance of, 66
Intensive courses, tips and techniques
    for, 186–188
Interaction with students, 145, 148, 152
Interactive activities, 66
Interactive approach, 165
International students, 45, 116
Interviews
    Billings, Diane M., 3–8
    Donley, Rosemary, Sister, 9–19
    Downs, Florence S., 20–29
    Ferguson, Vernice, 30–37
    Fitzpatrick, Joyce J., 171–175
    Fitzpatrick, M. Louise, 38–47
    Holzemer, William L., 48–55
    Ironside, Pamela, 56–61
    Jeffries, Pamela R., 62–69

Interviews (*continued*)
   Liehr, Patricia R., 70–76
   McBride, Angela Barron, 87–98
   Martin, E. Jane, 77–86
   Morris, Diana Lynn, 99–106
   Nyamathi, Adeline, 107–112
   Oermann, Marilyn, 113–117
   Rew, Lynn, 118–125
   Sills, Grayce M., 126–133
   Springer, Ursula, 134–138
   Tanner, Christine A., 139–148
   Tufts, Kimberly Adams, 149–155
   Van Ort, Suzanne, 156–162
   Wykle, May L., 163–170
Ironside, Pamela
   advice for new teachers, 61
   appointments, 56
   challenges faced, 59
   early interest in teaching, 57
   educational background, 56
   embarrassing moments, 60
   evolution as a teacher, 58–59
   feeling comfortable, 59
   least rewarding aspects of teaching, 60
   maintaining excellence, 60–61
   mentoring, 58
   preparation for teaching, 57–58
   professional background, 56
   professional memberships, 56
   rewarding aspects of teaching, 60

Jeffries, Pamela R.
   advice for new teachers, 68–69
   awards and recognitions, 67
   challenges faced, 66
   early interest in teaching, 63
   educational background, 62
   embarrassing moments, 66–67
   evolution as a teacher, 64–65
   feeling comfortable, 65
   least rewarding aspects of teaching, 68
   maintaining excellence, 68
   mentoring, 62–64
   preparation for teaching, 63
   professional background, 62
   rewarding aspects of teaching, 67–68
Johnson, Jean, 88

Kaplan, Gerald, 166
Knowles, Malcom, 151
Kramer, Marlene, 140, 142
Kramer, Mary Albert, Sister, 114
Kreigh, Helen, 164–165

Labadie, Georgie, 41–42, 44
Laidig, Juanita, Dr., 64
Lambertsen, Eleanor, 41
Language skills, 36
Leadership skills, 31
Learning environment, 26, 54, 90, 161
Learning process, 133
Learning styles, 153
Lecture development, 66
Leininger, Madeleine, 115–116
Liehr, Patricia R.
   advice for new teachers, 75–76
   challenges faced, 73
   early interest in teaching, 71
   educational background, 70
   embarrassing moments, 74
   evolution as a teacher, 72
   feeling comfortable, 72–73
   least rewarding aspects of teaching, 74–75
   maintaining excellence, 75
   mentoring, 71–72
   preparation for teaching, 71
   professional background, 70
   rewarding aspects of teaching, 74
Life associations, 164, 166
Lindeman, Carol, 143
Listening skills, 61, 68–69, 72, 91, 105, 148, 162
Literature review, 92

McBride, Angela Barron
   advice for new teachers, 97–98
   awards and recognitions, 87
   challenges faced, 93–94
   doctoral course, 15-credit, 91–93
   early interest in teaching, 88
   educational background, 87
   embarrassing moments, 94
   evolution as a teacher, 90–91

feeling comfortable, 93
least rewarding aspects of teaching, 95
maintaining excellence, 95–97
mentoring, 64, 89–90
preparation for teaching, 88–89
professional background, 5, 87
rewarding aspects of teaching, 94–95
Malone, Alice, 12–13, 18
Managed care, 15
Markle, Rebecca, 5
Marsell, James, 127
Martin, E. Jane
    advice for new teachers, 85–86
    challenges, 82–83
    early interest in teaching, 78–79
    educational background, 77
    embarrassing moments, 83
    feeling comfortable, 82
    least rewarding aspects of teaching,
        85
    maintaining excellence, 85
    mentoring, 79–82
    preparation for teaching, 79
    professional background, 77
    professional memberships, 77
    rewarding aspects of teaching, 84
Master's programs, 10–11, 18
Meaningful advice, types of, 201–203
Media, instructional, 68
Medical education, 55
Mentors/mentoring, impact of, 5, 14, 20,
        22, 28–29, 32, 41–42, 46, 49–50,
        58, 62–64, 71–72, 79–82, 89–90,
        102, 108, 114–115, 117–118,
        121–122, 128–129, 134, 142, 151,
        155, 158, 164–165, 172–173
Mereness, Dorothy, 164–165
Miraldo, Pam, 143
Moccia, Pat, 143
Montag, Mildred, 40–41, 127
Moral authority, 95
Morris, Diana Lynn
    advice for new teachers, 106
    awards and recognitions, 99
    challenges faced, 104
    early interest in teaching, 100–101
    educational background, 99

embarrassing moments, 104
evolution as a teacher, 102–103
feeling comfortable, 103
least rewarding aspects of teaching,
    105
maintaining excellence, 105–106
mentoring, 102
preparation for teaching, 101–102
professional background, 99
rewarding aspects of teaching,
    104–105
Motivation, importance of, 34
Mullane, Mary Kelly, Dr., 36
Murphy, John, Dr., 14
Murray, Joyce, 143

National Research Service Award
    (NRSA), 73
Networking, 175
New teachers, advice for, 8, 18–19,
        28–29, 36–37, 46–47, 53–55, 61,
        68–69, 75–76, 85–86, 97–98, 106,
        111–112, 117, 125, 133, 147–148,
        154–155, 161–162, 169–170;
    see also Tips and techniques
Nonstructured classes, 59
Nurse administrator, functions of, 36;
    see also Administrative functions
Nurse–patient relationship, 168
Nurse scientists, 160
Nursing history, 40
Nursing research, 69
Nutting, Adelaide, 40
Nyamathi, Adeline
    administrative functions, 107
    advice for new teachers, 111–112
    challenges faced, 110
    early interest in teaching, 108
    educational background, 107
    embarrassing moments, 110
    evolution as a teacher, 108–110
    feeling comfortable, 110
    least rewarding aspects of teaching,
        111
    maintaining excellence, 111
    mentoring, 108
    preparation for teaching, 108

Nyamathi, Adeline *(continued)*
  professional background, 107
  professional memberships, 107
  rewarding aspects of teaching, 110

Oermann, Marilyn
  advice for new teachers, 117
  challenges faced, 115
  early interest in teaching, 114
  educational background, 113
  embarrassing moments, 115–116
  evolution as a teacher, 115
  feeling comfortable, 115
  least rewarding aspects of teaching,
    116
  maintaining excellence, 117
  mentoring, 114–115, 117
  preparation for teaching, 114
  professional background, 113
  rewarding aspects of teaching, 116
On-line courses, 65, 69, 116–117
On-line environment, 6
Organizational structure, 6–7
Other-regarding approach, 181

Partnership, teacher/learner, 154–155
Passion, importance of, 36; *see also*
    Enthusiasm
Patient education, 22, 165–166
Patient Education and Counseling,
    120
Pedagogical approach, 58
Pellegrino, Edmund, Dr., 13–14
Peplau, Hildegard, 128–131, 165, 172
Person-centered teaching, 122
Phipps, Wilma, Dr., 151
Political structure, 7
Potential development, 25–26, 35–36
Process recordings, 89, 93
Psychiatric nursing, 11, 22–23, 25,
    81, 85

Quality care, 100–101, 113
Quality monitoring, 147
Questioning/questions
  dialogue engagement, 178–179, 181
  response to, 75–76

Socratic, 24, 72, 178–179
  use of, 59, 72

Reading, importance of, 35–37, 68, 85
Reflective thinking, 89
Reilly, Dorothy, 114–115
Relationship nursing, 165
Research, generally
  competence, 41
  importance of, 61
  intensive environments, 54
  skills, 47
  socialization, 96
Research courses, 197–201
Research instructors, 22–23
Resnick, Michael, 121–122
Responsibility, 82; *see also*
    Accountability; Ethical
    responsibility
Rew, Lynn
  advice for new teachers, 125
  challenges faced, 123
  early interest in teaching, 119
  educational background, 118
  embarrassing moments, 123
  evolution as a teacher, 122
  feeling comfortable, 122–123
  maintaining excellence, 124–125
  mentoring, 118, 121–122
  preparation for teaching, 119–120
  professional background, 118
  rewarding aspects of teaching, 124
Risk-taking, 174
Rogers, Martha, 22, 24, 121, 173

Scales, Freda, Dr., 63
Schaefer, Marguerite, Dr., 79–80
Schlotfeldt, Rozella, 36
Scholarship environment, 54
Schulman, Lee, 147
Self-awareness, 105, 148
Self-consciousness, 90
Self-evaluation, 69
Self-illumination, 181
Self-in-relation, 70
Seminars, benefits of, 164, 169
Shaeffer, Frank, 143

Sharp, Elizabeth, 88
Shiloh, Ahlon, Dr., 11–12
Sills, Grayce M.
    advice for new teachers, 133
    awards and recognitions, 126
    challenges faced, 131
    early interest in teaching, 127
    educational background, 126
    embarrasing moments, 131–132
    evolution as a teacher, 129–130
    feeling comfortable, 130–131
    least rewarding aspects of teaching,
        132–133
    maintaining excellence, 133
    mentoring, 128–129, 172–173
    preparation for teaching, 127–128
    professional background, 126
    professional memberships, 126
    rewarding aspects of teaching, 132
Sindlinger, Walter, 41
Smith, Mary Jane
    interest in teaching, 177
    story-moments, 176, 178–179
    teaching/learning sessions, 180–181
    trust development, 179–180
Smoyak, Shirley, 132
Society for Research in Nursing
        Education, 54, 142–143
Socratic method, 24, 72, 178–179
Sorensen, Gladys, Dr., 158
Specialties, selection of, 59
Springer, Ursula
    awards and recognitions, 134
    challenges faced, 137
    early interest in teaching, 135–138
    educational background, 134–135
    embarrasing moments, 137
    evolution as a teacher, 137
    mentoring, 134
    professional background, 134–136
Staff development, 119–120
Stereotypes, 97, 167
Stokes, Lillian, 5
Story theory, 70
Student anxiety, dealing with, 168–169
Student behavior
    advice for new teachers, 111

angry students, 76
disruptive students, 111, 137
failure, 35, 66, 137
hostile students, 111
response to, 76
successful students, 174
Student-centered approach, 60, 62, 64–65
Student development, 170
Student engagement, 58–59, 89, 101,
        140, 146–147
Student growth, 104–105, 110, 154
Student learning, 148
Student population, generational differ-
        ences in, 145
Successful students, characteristics of, 174
Support system, 46

Tanner, Christine A.
    advice for new teachers, 147–148
    challenges faced, 145–146
    curriculum development, 139
    early interest in teaching, 140
    educational background, 139
    embarrasing moments, 146
    evolution as a teacher, 142–144
    feeling comfortable, 145
    fellowships, 139
    least rewarding aspects of teaching,
        147
    maintaining excellence, 147
    mentoring, 142
    preparation for teaching, 140–142
    professional background, 139
    rewarding aspects of teaching,
        146–147
Teacher-centered approach, 64–65
Teacher-scientist, 55
Teacher–student relationship, 26, 48–49,
        58, 85, 128, 145, 152, 166, 168,
        178–179
Teaching approaches/methods, 22
Teaching style, development of, 5–6,
        12–15, 22–24, 32–33, 42–44,
        50–51, 58–59, 64–65, 72, 90–91,
        102–103, 108–110, 115, 128–130,
        137, 142–144, 151–152, 158,
        165–166

Teaching-learning process, 170
Teaching-learning theory, 153–154
Team teaching, 124
Technological advances, impact of, 6, 46,
    53, 55
Tenure, 117, 159
Time management, 73, 82–83, 93–94, 174
Tips and techniques
    clinical courses, 188–194
    distance education courses, 194–197
    intensive courses, 186–188
    meaningful advice, types of, 201–203
    research courses, 197–201
    for undergraduate teaching, 185
    "what if" questions, 184
    writing exercises, 184
Tufts, Kimberly Adams
    advice for new teachers, 154–155
    challenges faced, 152–153
    early interest in teaching, 150
    educational background, 149
    embarrassing moments, 153
    evolution as a teacher, 151–152
    feeling comfortable, 152
    least rewarding aspects of teaching, 154
    maintaining excellence, 154
    mentoring, 151, 155
    preparation for teaching, 150–151
    professional background, 149
    rewarding aspects of teaching,
        153–154
    student-centered approach, 149

Undergraduate teaching, 7 principles for,
    185

Valanis, Barbara, 144
Van Ort, Suzanne
    advice for new teachers, 161–162
    awards and recognitions, 156
    challenges faced, 159–160
    early interest in teaching, 157
    educational background, 156

evolution of teaching, 158
feeling comfortable, 159
least rewarding aspects of teaching,
    160–161
maintaining excellence, 161
mentoring, 158
preparation for teaching, 157–158
professional background, 156
professional fellowships, 156
rewarding aspects of teaching, 160
teacher–student relationship,
    156–157
Vocational nursing programs, 33

Walton, Clarence, Dr., 13
Watson, Jean, 143
Websites, as information resource, 97;
    see also On-line courses
Werley, Harriet, 173
Wiedenbach, Ernestine, 88
Workshops, benefits of, 68, 100–101,
    103, 117
Wright, Helen, 102
Writing exercises, personal biography,
    184
Wykle, May L.
    advice for new teachers, 169–170
    awards and recognitions, 163
    challenges faced, 166–167
    early interest in teaching, 164
    educational background, 163
    embarrrassing moments,
        167–168
    evolution as a teacher, 165–166
    feeling comfortable, 166
    least rewarding aspects of teaching,
        168–169
    life associations, 164, 166
    mentoring, 102, 164–165
    preparation for teaching, 164
    professional background, 163
    rewarding aspects of teaching,
        168